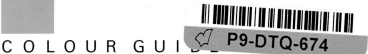

COLOUR GUIDE

Dermatology

J.D. Wilkinson MB BS MRCS FRCP
Consultant Dermatologist, Wycombe General Hospital,
High Wycombe, UK

S. Shaw MB ChB MRCP
Associate Specialist in Dermatology,
Wycombe General Hospital, High Wycombe, UK

D.A. Fenton MB ChB MRCS MRCP
Senior Registrar in Dermatology,
St Thomas's Hospital, London, UK

Churchill Livingstone

EDINBURGH LONDON MADRID MELBOURNE NEW YORK AND TOKYO 1993

Acknowledgements

We would like to acknowledge the expert assistance of Alison Carter and Rosemary May, Department of Medical Illustration, Wycombe General Hospital. We also extend our thanks to the Department of Dermatology, The Slade Hospital, Oxford, for their permission to reproduce illustrations borrowed from their collection.

High Wycombe and London,   J.D.W.
1993   S.S.
                                                           D.A.F.

Contents

1 / Benign childhood pigmented naevi

Freckles

Aetiology Increased activity of melanocytes.

Clinical features Brown macules (usually in redheads). They appear in early childhood, and darken on sun exposure (Fig. 1).

Treatment Sunscreens and/or sun protection.

Lentigo

Aetiology A localized proliferation of melanocytes.

Clinical features Areas of brown or black pigmentation, usually 1–2 mm in diameter. These appear in childhood but may proliferate in adulthood. They do not darken or proliferate on sun exposure (Fig. 2).

Treatment None. However, a solitary lentigo appearing in adult life and continuing to grow may be a malignant melanoma.

Pigmented naevus/birthmark

Aetiology Developmental defect.

Clinical features Localized pigmented and sometimes hairy naevus (Fig. 3), present from birth, up to 2–3 cm in size. Giant hairy naevus is a rare developmental defect with a potential for malignant transformation. Surgical excision should be considered.

Treatment None; excision if required.

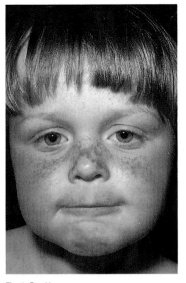

Fig. 1 Freckles.

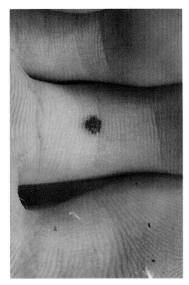

Fig. 2 Lentigo.

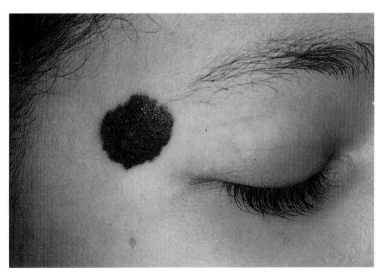

Fig. 3 Pigmented birthmark.

Cellular naevus

Synonym Melanocytic/pigmented naevus or mole.

Aetiology Developmental defect. Melanocyte proliferation occurs at the dermo-epidermal junction or in the dermis.

Clinical features Not normally present at birth, but develops during childhood, particularly at puberty. It may enlarge or darken during pregnancy, and may be pink, brown or black, flat or raised, hairy or non-hairy (Figs 4 & 5). Blue naevus (Fig. 6) is a variant with dermal pigmentation. Malignant transformation is possible in those with large numbers of pigmented naevi or 'atypical' moles and a family history of melanoma.

Treatment Excision only in the case of frequent trauma or malignant transformation. All excised moles should be submitted for histology.

Juvenile melanoma (benign)

Synonym Spitz naevus.

Aetiology A variant of cellular naevus.

Clinical features A solitary, reddish-brown nodule occurring in childhood (usually affecting the face), growing rapidly to 1 cm. The lesion is benign, although the histology may resemble malignant melanoma (Fig. 7).

Treatment None or simple excision.

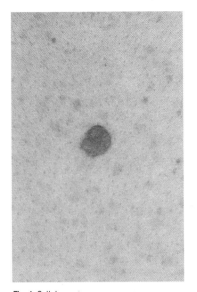

Fig. 4 Cellular naevus.

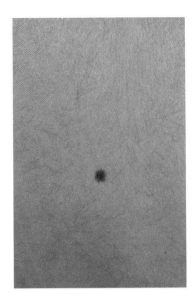

Fig. 5 Pigmented cellular naevus.

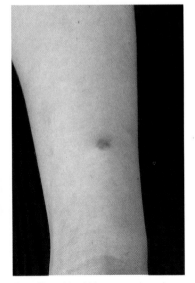

Fig. 6 Blue rubber-bleb naevus.

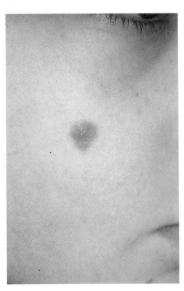

Fig. 7 Juvenile melanoma (Spitz naevus).

2 / Genodermatoses

Peutz-Jeghers syndrome

Synonym Periorificial lentiginosis.

Aetiology Rare autosomal dominant inherited disorder.

Clinical features Blue-brown macules affect the buccal mucosa, gums, lips (Fig. 8), palate, palms and soles. Lentigines are obvious either at, or soon after, birth. The condition is associated with small intestinal polyps. These may cause recurrent intussusception or ulcerate and lead to haemorrhage. Malignant transformation of polyps may occur but is rare.

Treatment The lentigines require no therapy.

Neurofibromatosis

Synonym von Recklinghausen's disease.

Aetiology An autosomal dominant inherited condition with approximately 50% rate of new mutations.

Clinical features Characterised by multiple, light brown, 'café-au-lait', macular patches of several cm diameter (Fig. 9). Some may be present from birth. There may also be axillary freckling (Fig. 10). The skin neurofibromas which develop as the child grows up are soft, dome-shaped, pedunculated or plexiform. They vary in number from a few to hundreds (Fig. 11). Size also varies from a few mm to enormous plexiform neuromas with hypertrophy of the subcutaneous tissues and skin. Systemic manifestations include kyphosis, scoliosis, bone cysts, phaeochromocytoma, acromegaly, acoustic neuroma, glioma and mental deficiency.

Treatment Genetic counselling; excision of symptomatic neurofibromas.

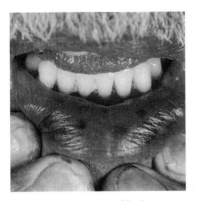

Fig. 8 Macular pigmentation of lips in Peutz-Jeghers syndrome.

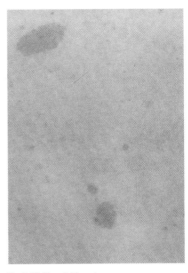

Fig. 9 'Café-au-lait' spots.

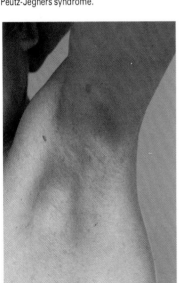

Fig. 10 Axillary freckling.

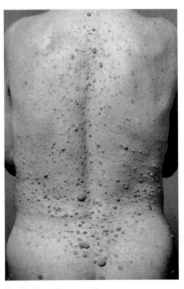

Fig. 11 Neurofibromatosis.

Tuberous sclerosis

Synonym	Epiloia.
Aetiology	Autosomal dominant condition of skin and CNS.
Clinical features	Depigmented 'ash-leaf'-shaped macules occur on the trunk and limbs, varying in size from a few mm to a few cm. They may be more obvious under Wood's light (Fig. 12). There is no treatment. Other characteristic lesions present are as follows.

Adenoma sebaceum

Clinical features Cutaneous angiofibromata produce small discrete pink papules affecting mainly the central face (Fig. 13). They are not present at birth but appear within the first few years of life. They can be confused with acne.

Treatment Diathermy, dermabrasion or CO_2 or argon laser.

Periungual fibromas

Clinical features Firm, smooth, filiform tumours emerging from the base of the nails (Fig. 14).

Treatment None. Excision or diathermy.

Shagreen patches (collagen naevi)

Clinical features Skin coloured/yellowish plaques occurring on the trunk.

Treatment None.

Fig. 12 'Ash-leaf' spot.

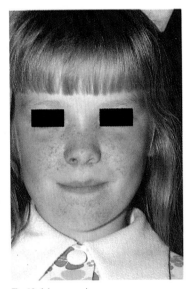

Fig. 13 Adenoma sebaceum.

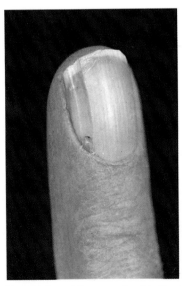

Fig. 14 Periungual fibroma causing distortion of nail plate.

Ehlers-Danlos syndrome

Aetiology A rare group of inherited collagen disorders.

Clinical features The skin is characteristically soft, doughy and hyperextensible, the joints are hypermobile or 'double-jointed' (Fig. 15). Cutis laxa may occur (Fig. 16). The skin is fragile and bruises easily; scars are atrophic and wide (Fig. 17). The sclerae are blue.

Treatment No specific therapy, but lacerations/injuries require specialist attention to minimize scarring.

Pseudoxanthoma elasticum

Aetiology Rare inherited disorder of elastic tissue.

Clinical features Distinctive skin lesions, retinal changes and vascular disturbances. The skin is soft, lax and wrinkled with yellowish papules in a reticulate pattern or in plaques, giving the appearance of chicken skin or 'peau d'orange'. The sides of the neck, axillae and anticubital fossae are characteristically affected (Fig. 18). Slate-grey angioid streaks are seen on the retina. Arterial involvement may cause haemorrhage from the gut or elsewhere. Hypertension is also common.

Treatment Avoid traumatic sports/hobbies or occupations which may lead to eye damage.

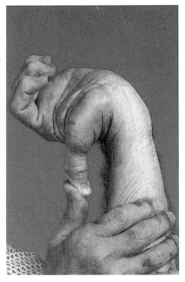

Fig. 15 Hyperextensible joint (Ehlers-Danlos).

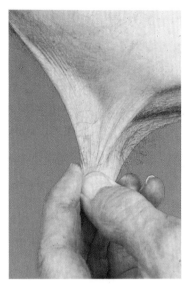

Fig. 16 Cutis laxa (Ehlers-Danlos).

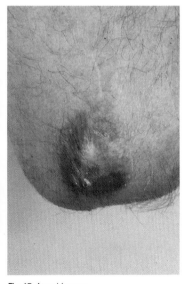

Fig. 17 Atrophic scar.

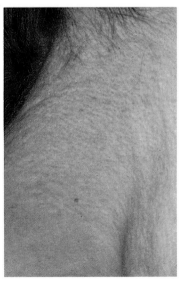

Fig. 18 Peau d'orange (PXE).

3 / Benign childhood vascular tumours

Portwine stain (capillary haemangioma)

Aetiology   Developmental defect of mature dermal capillaries.

Clinical features   An erythematous or purplish macular naevus (Fig. 19) present at birth. It is usually unilateral, affecting face, trunk or limb, and variable in size. It may be associated with underlying arteriovenous malformation. Limb involvement may result in hypertrophy (Klippel-Trenaunay syndrome); a capillary naevus in the trigeminal area may be part of the Sturge-Weber syndrome.

Treatment   Cosmetic camouflage; argon or tuneable dye laser may help.

Strawberry naevus (cavernous haemangioma)

Aetiology   Developmental; benign angioblastic proliferation.

Clinical features   Develops rapidly during the first 6 months of life. It is a well-demarcated, compressible vascular swelling (Figs 20 & 21) that normally undergoes spontaneous resolution. Haemorrhage, ulceration and thrombocytopenia are rare complications.

Treatment   None—spontaneous resolution. Surgery may be necessary for redundant folds of skin. High dose steroids are (rarely) given if severe thrombocytopenia, cardiac failure, or vital functions are affected.

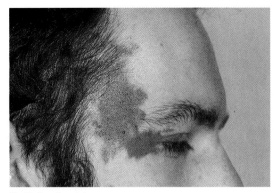

Fig. 19 Portwine stain.

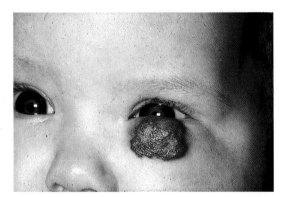

Fig. 20 Strawberry naevus.

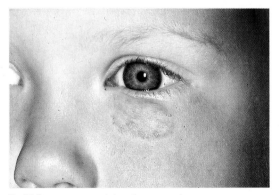

Fig. 21 Spontaneous resolution of same strawberry naevus.

Spider naevus

Aetiology A small, superficial arteriole giving rise to a localized telangiectasia.

Clinical features A central, raised, erythematous papule with radiating dilated capillaries. Lesions commonly occur on the face (Fig. 22), and often proliferate during pregnancy or liver disease. If lesions are multiple and involve mucosal surfaces, hereditary haemorrhagic telangiectasia should be considered.

Treatment 'Cold-point' cautery or 'epilating' electrodiathermy to the central arteriole.

Salmon patch

Aetiology A localized, capillary, telangiectatic naevus.

Clinical features A pale pink area, commonly found in newborn infants on the nape of the neck, glabella or over one eye (Fig. 23). No treatment is required.

Pyogenic granuloma

Aetiology Abnormal proliferation of capillaries following trauma or infection.

Clinical features A friable and often pedunculated vascular nodule (Fig. 24), bleeding easily and profusely when traumatized.

Treatment Curettage and cautery under local anaesthetic. In adults, histology is necessary since the lesion can be confused with amelanotic malignant melanoma.

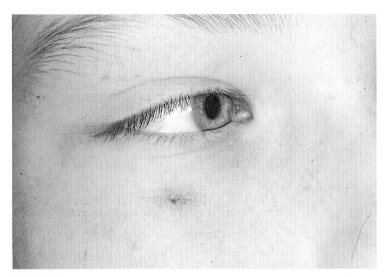

Fig. 22 Spider naevus.

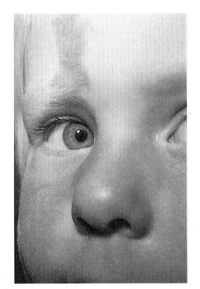

Fig. 23 Salmon patch. Facial lesions fade but those on nape of neck may persist.

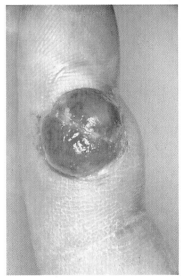

Fig. 24 Pyogenic granuloma. Grows rapidly, commonly affecting areas of trauma.

4 / Napkin eruptions

Napkin candidiasis

Aetiology   Yeast infection with *Candida albicans*.

Clinical features   Well-demarcated erythema with scaling extending from the perineum, normally involving the skin folds. There may be isolated 'satellite' lesions and/or pustules. Oral lesions and intertriginous infections are common (Figs 25 & 26) (see also p. 135).

Treatment   Swabs; nystatin and imidazole creams (or a hydrocortisone/imidazole or antiseptic combination); reduction of occlusion and eradication of yeast carriage. An appropriate dusting powder may prevent relapse.

Napkin psoriasis

Aetiology   Local factors; possible genetic predisposition.

Clinical features   Develops suddenly, normally at about 4–8 weeks. Dark-red and scaly lesions with well-defined margins are seen in the napkin area (Fig. 27) and often on the scalp. Smaller scattered lesions can develop elsewhere on the trunk. Napkin area lesions are larger, asymptomatic and may extend to the flexures. Often clears spontaneously within a few weeks.

Treatment   Bland applications and mild topical steroids or steroid/antiseptic combinations.

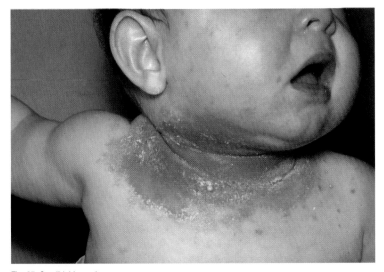

Fig. 25 Candidal intertrigo.

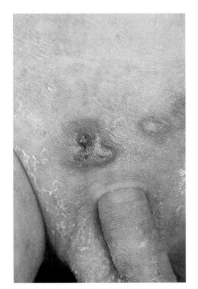

Fig. 26 Granuloma gluteale infantum (*Candida*).

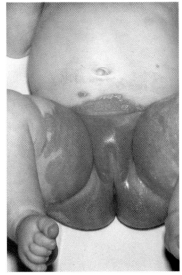

Fig. 27 Psoriasiform napkin rash.

Seborrhoeic eczema

Aetiology Unknown. Constitutional and microbial factors may coexist.

Clinical features Appearance at 2–10 weeks. Asymptomatic, well-defined, round or oval patches of erythema and greasy scaling extend to form gyrate patterns in the genitocrural flexures. Scalp, ears and other body folds may be involved (Fig. 28).

Treatment Cleansing cream and mild topical steroid/antiseptic.

Napkin dermatitis

Aetiology Inflammatory disorder produced by prolonged contact with urine, faeces or irritant chemicals in napkin. It may be the first manifestation of atopic eczema.

Clinical features Genitalia, buttocks, lower abdomen and upper thighs are affected. Flexures are normally spared (Fig. 29). Initial erythema, but vesicles, papules, erosions and ulcers may develop. Fine scaling with glazed erythema is seen in chronic forms.

Treatment Emollients and weak topical steroids. Frequent changing and thorough cleaning with a mild non-soap cleanser e.g. aqueous cream. Plastic napkins/pants should be avoided and nappies left off where possible. A barrier cream can be used at night. Candidiasis or secondary bacterial infections should be treated appropriately.

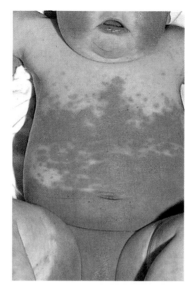

Fig. 28 Seborrhoeic dermatitis of infants.

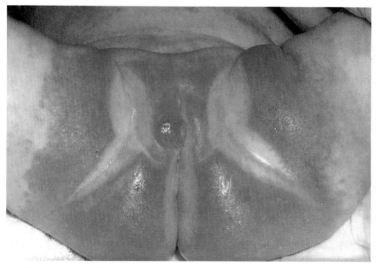

Fig. 29 Ammoniacal napkin rash.

5 / Atopic eczema

Asthma, hay fever and infantile eczema tend to run in families. Up to 25% of the population are potentially 'atopic', although less than 10% develop eczema.

Synonym Infantile eczema.

Aetiology Inheritance of atopic diathesis; sensitivity/allergy to foreign proteins (type I hypersensitivity reactions); a generally intolerant and vulnerable ('leaky') skin. Eczema is made worse by cold (low humidity), heat, woollen clothing, infections and stress.

Clinical features Atopic eczema can occur at any age, but often develops about 3 months after birth. Intense pruritus is a prominent feature (Fig. 30).

Facial: the face is often involved in babies (Fig. 31). Itchy, erythematous papules on the cheeks or erythematosquamous dry/'chapped' or hypopigmented areas may be seen. Infraorbital lines (Morgan's folds) are common in atopic individuals.

Flexural: characteristic in early childhood. There is symmetrical involvement of elbow and knee flexures, wrists and ankles. The skin is generally dry and lichenified or excoriated. Constant licking of lips in some children causes 'lick eczema' (Fig. 32).

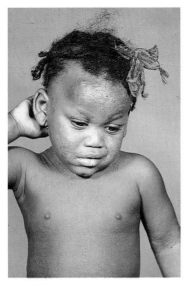

Fig. 30 Childhood atopic eczema.

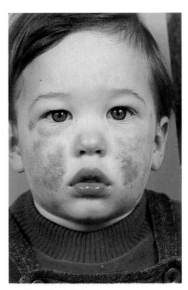

Fig. 31 Facial atopic eczema.

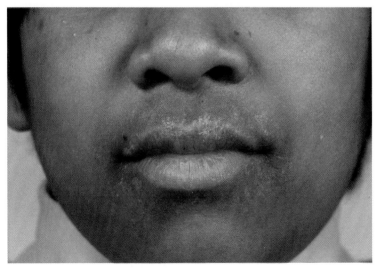

Fig. 32 'Lick eczema'.

Clinical features
(cont)

Reverse pattern: the extensor surfaces of arms and legs are involved in some children. The pattern of eczema in these cases is frequently 'discoid' (Fig. 33). A 'papular' form of eczema is common in Negroes. (Fig. 34).

Lichenification: constant rubbing and scratching gives rise to areas of thickened skin with increased skin markings. This is particularly seen around flexures (Fig. 35).

Secondary infection: this is common and may both exacerbate eczema and produce local lymphadenopathy (Fig. 37, p. 24).

Eczema herpeticum: herpes simplex (and in the past vaccinia) may disseminate widely in patients with atopic eczema (Fig. 38, p. 24). Viral warts and molluscum contagiosum also occur more commonly in atopics.

Superficial, hypopigmented: patches of eczema affecting the face in children (Fig. 36) (*pityriasis alba*) and/or trunk and limbs. It is not necessarily always associated with atopy. The condition is often more active in winter (low humidity), but more obvious in summer. It is poorly responsive to treatment but will improve with time. Emollients may help.

Juvenile plantar dermatosis (forefoot eczema): frictional and occlusive factors are important in this condition as it seems to be a result of modern footwear. Atopics may be more susceptible. The feet have a characteristic glazed appearance with dryness and fissures (Fig. 39, p. 24).

'Nappy rash': primary irritant napkin dermatitis may occasionally be the first manifestation of atopic eczema (see also p. 19).

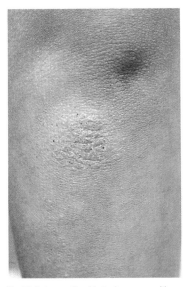

Fig. 33 Extensor discoid atopic eczema with post-inflammatory hypopigmentation.

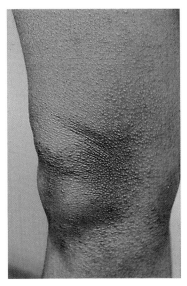

Fig. 34 Follicular/papular eczema.

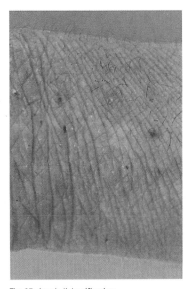

Fig. 35 Atopic lichenification.

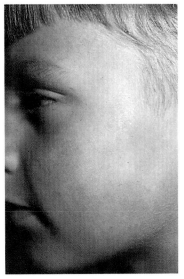

Fig. 36 Pityriasis alba (chronic superficial depigmenting dermatitis).

Treatment

Soap substitutes and water softeners/bath emollients: aqueous creams, oatmeal preparations and bath oils should be used.

Emollients: E45 cream, oily cream and simple ointment need to be used frequently to help hydrate the skin.

Tar preparations: Coal tar paste or coal tar paste bandages are useful in chronic or lichenified eczema (applied on top of steroid).

Topical steroids: extremely effective. The potency of steroids used will depend on age, extent and activity of eczema. In general, hydrocortisone is preferred for children and facial/flexural skin, but short bursts of stronger steroids may be required to bring eczema under control.

Topical antibiotics: may be required for infected eczema; these are often combined with a topical steroid. Systemic antibiotics are also often necessary.

Sedative antihistamines: help to reduce pruritus, especially at night.

Cotton clothing: preferable as wool causes itching.

Wet compresses: very helpful in the initial management of acute eczema.

Systemic acyclovir: often required for eczema herpeticum, which is a medical emergency.

Counselling: about the possible role of house dust mite, dietary factors, etc. should be given to parents, and children should be given career advice so as to avoid irritant and wet work.

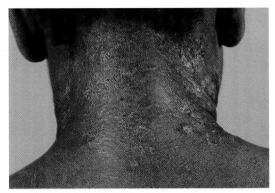

Fig. 37 Secondarily infected atopic eczema.

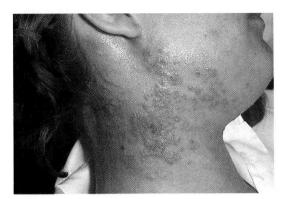

Fig. 38 Extensive herpes simplex in an atopic.

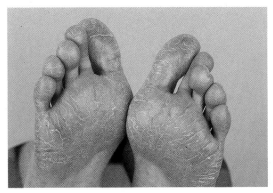

Fig. 39 Juvenile plantar dermatosis. The result of friction and occlusive footwear.

6 / Childhood scalp conditions

Tinea/pityriasis amiantacea

Aetiology Distinctive reaction pattern of scalp. It may be associated with psoriasis/eczema.

Clinical features Asbestos-like, silvery scales adhere firmly to scalp and hair (Fig. 40). If there is associated infection the underlying scalp is erythematous and moist. There may be some loss of hair.

Treatment 1–2% salicylic acid in arachis oil or aqueous cream, tar-containing keratolytic preparations such as Cocois with tar shampoos, steroid/antibacterial creams. Occasionally systemic antibiotics and stronger tar preparations may be needed.

Cradle cap (seborrhoeic eczema)

Aetiology Unknown; possible constitutional and microbial factors.

Clinical features Appears at 0–3 months. The scalp is covered with 'greasy' scales (Fig. 41). The cheeks, flexures of neck, axillae, napkin areas and ears are often affected. It may mimic psoriasis.

Treatment Mild keratolytics, e.g. 2% salicylic acid in arachis oil for the scalp; non-soap cleansers and hydrocortisone-antiseptic combinations elsewhere.

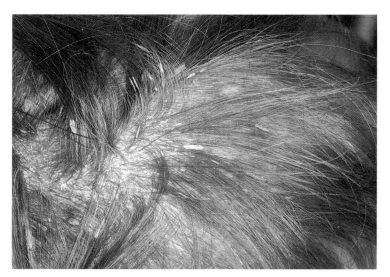

Fig. 40 Tinea amiantacea.

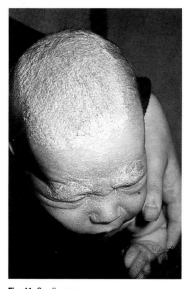

Fig. 41 Cradle cap.

Ringworm

Synonym   Tinea capitis.

Aetiology   *Microsporum audouinii* and *M. canis* invade hair shafts. The former condition is now, fortunately, a rarity. *M. canis* is, however, commonly contracted from cats and dogs (especially puppies). Animal trichophyton infections cause more severe reactions.

Clinical features   The condition is usually seen in children and produces circular, erythematous bald patches with scaling and broken hair shafts (Fig. 42). Wood's light examination shows a green/blue fluorescence for *M. audouinii* or *M. canis* (Fig. 43), but not for other types of fungus. A more inflammatory reaction follows infection with animal ringworm (cows, horses, etc.) (Fig. 44). This produces a tender and much more pustular *kerion* (Fig. 45). This may ultimately cause scarring alopecia. Fungal microscopy and culture is usually positive, but false-negative results may occur with kerion.

Treatment   Oral griseofulvin is the treatment of choice. The affected hair should be 'cropped' short and treatment continued for at least 6 weeks. Topical antifungal agents may also be used. Several new oral antifungal drugs are now also available.

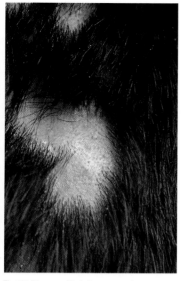

Fig. 42 Tinea capitis (microsporum).

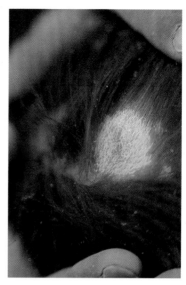

Fig. 43 Characteristic green/blue fluorescence under Wood's light.

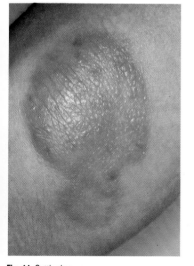

Fig. 44 Cattle ringworm.

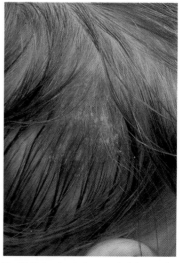

Fig. 45 Kerion (cattle ringworm) of the scalp.

7 / Childhood bacterial infections

Impetigo

Aetiology

A contagious superficial skin infection caused by staphylococci and/or β-haemolytic streptococci.

Clinical features

Bullae may rupture to produce golden-yellow crusts (Fig. 46). The disease can become epidemic in over-crowded conditions. Scabies, lice and eczema predispose. Glomerulonephritis may be a rare complication (strep.).

Treatment

Swabs followed by topical or systemic antibiotics. Staphylococcal or streptococcal carriage should be eradicated from nose (staph.), throat (strep.), and perineum (both) (Fig. 47). Close family members should be screened.

Infantile toxic epidermal necrolysis

Aetiology

Staphylococci (usually phage type 71) liberate toxins leading to large superficial erosions (Fig. 47). Drugs may produce a similar syndrome in adults.

Clinical features

A rare disease following minor skin infections or impetigo in infants. The process mimics a burn or scald (Fig. 48). Untreated, the disease may be fatal.

Treatment

Swabs followed by appropriate systemic antibiotic therapy. Dehydration and electrolyte imbalance should be corrected. Treat topically, as for burns.

Toxic shock syndrome

Aetiology

Toxin produced by focal phage group I (usually penicillin-resistant) staphylococcal infection.

Clinical features

Fever, diarrhoea, shock and erythematous rash.

Treatment

General supportive measures. Penicillinase-resistant antibiotic therapy.

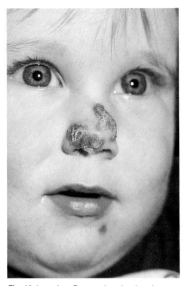

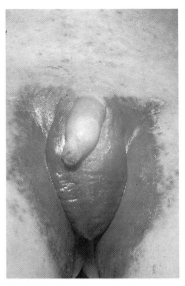

Fig. 46 Impetigo. Face and perioral region are frequently affected.

Fig. 47 Mixed staphylococcal and streptoccal intertrigo.

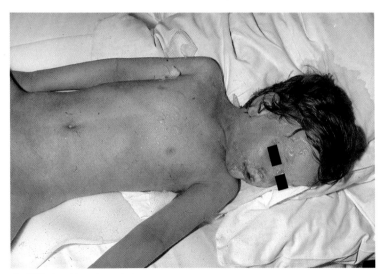

Fig. 48 Toxic epidermal necrolysis.

8 / Childhood viral infections

Warts

Aetiology Reactive epidermal proliferation caused by infection with human papilloma virus.

Common wart
Clinical features Elevated, hyperkeratotic papules with a rough surface occurring mainly on the hands (Fig. 50) and knees. They are solitary or multiple and arise in areas of trauma (especially the nail fold in nail-biters and cuticle-pickers). Warts generally resolve spontaneously within 2 or 3 years and are not usually painful.

Treatment Depends on type, number, site, patient's determination. Proprietary wart paints containing salicylic acid or glutaraldehyde combined with regular pumice and occlusion may be effective, as may freezing with liquid N_2, NO_2 or CO_2 snow. (Several applications may be needed.) Rarely, curettage and cauterization is necessary.

Filiform warts
Clinical features Small digitate warts which often appear in clusters on the face (Fig. 49). In adults, shaving tends to cause them to spread.

Treatment Cryotherapy, superficial curettage and cauterization, diathermy. Podophyllin paint can be used if they are not too close to the eyes.

Plane warts
Clinical features Multiple smooth, small, flat-topped papules (Fig. 51) which may be linear or coalesce due to trauma (Koebner phenomenon) (Fig. 52, p. 34), occuring in young children and occasionally in adults. The face and backs of hands are particularly affected. They persist longer than other warts and respond less well to treatment. They will eventually disappear spontaneously.

Treatment 2% salicylic acid in 70% spirit lotion is usually adequate (as placebo).

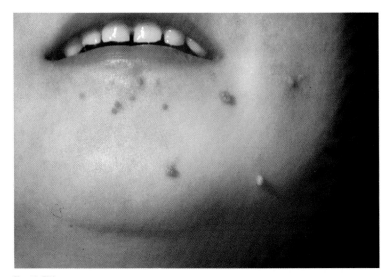

Fig. 49 Filiform warts.

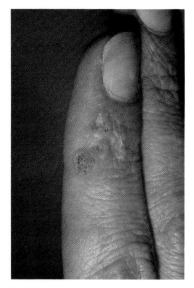

Fig. 50 Common warts.

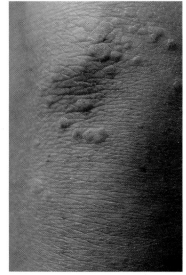

Fig. 51 Plane warts.

Plantar warts (verrucae)

Clinical features   Deep, hyperkeratotic, often tender lesions on the sole (Fig. 53). Body weight causes them to grow inwards rather than outwards. They are differentiated from corns/calluses by paring; warts have areas of black speckling and fine bleeding points. Multiple superficial plantar warts may coalesce to form a 'mosaic wart' which is very resistant to therapy and implies poor natural resistance (Fig. 54).

Treatment   Combination of paring and salicylic acid plasters or paints (under occlusion). Weekly applications of monochloracetic acid (caution: highly caustic) or intermittent treatment with liquid NO_2 can be effective. Therapy may be required for several weeks or months. Curettage and cautery may be employed for the occasional resistant verruca, but is painful even with local anaesthetic.

Genital warts (condyloma acuminata)

Aetiology   In children, infection may be associated with both genital and non-genital strains of human papilloma virus. Heteroinoculation and autoinoculation may both occur, and transmission may be both sexual and non-sexual.

Clinical features   Typically soft, pink, filiform or pedunculated affecting the glans and prepuce, vulva or perianal skin.

Treatment   A search for evidence of wart virus elsewhere and in other family members may reveal a potential source of infection. The possibility of sexual abuse and other sexually-transmitted disease should be kept in mind, but the majority of genital warts in children are probably not sexually transmitted. Treatment with intermittent topical 15% podophyllin, 0.5% podophyllotoxin and/or cryotherapy is usually successful.

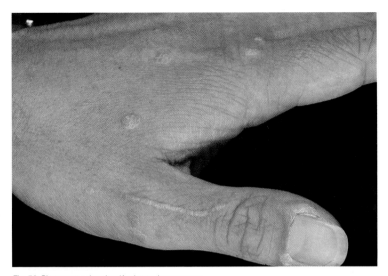

Fig. 52 Plane warts showing Koebner phenomenon.

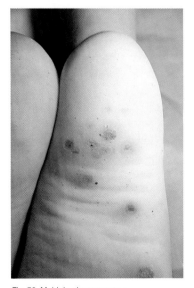

Fig. 53 Multiple plantar warts.

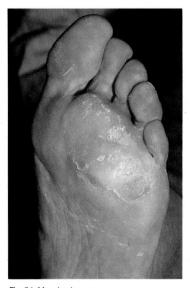

Fig. 54 Mosaic plantar wart.

Molluscum contagiosum

Aetiology   Pox virus.

Clinical features   Common in childhood, especially in atopics. Lesions are characteristically grouped, pearly white or pink, firm, umbilicated papules (Fig. 55) with a central depression and commonly affect the face, neck, trunk and perineum, although any area may be involved. They may grow to 5–10 mm in diameter if left untreated, and soften as they mature. Some become inflamed or secondarily infected.

Treatment   Lesions are easily removed with a sharp wooden cocktail stick or may be 'spiked' with phenol or iodine, or painted with podophyllin. They can also be removed by curettage, cryotherapy, diathermy or any other mildly traumatic procedure. Localized areas may be pre-treated with EMLA topical local anaesthetic and occlusion to facilitate treatment. Mollusca will however resolve spontaneously in time.

Hand, foot and mouth disease

Aetiology   A Coxsackie infection; epidemic. It mainly affects young children.

Clinical features   The disease is usually mild, with an incubation period of 5–7 days. There are scattered vesicles in the mouth and on the palms/soles (Fig. 56). Those in the mouth soon break down to leave small ulcers (Fig. 57). In some children there may be a more widespread exanthem.

Treatment   None.

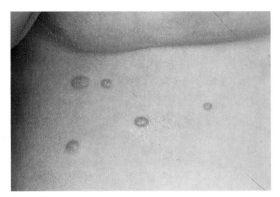

Fig. 55 Molluscum contagiosum.

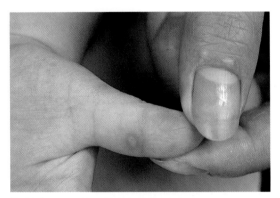

Fig. 56 Characteristic vesicle in hand, foot and mouth disease.

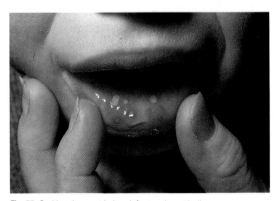

Fig. 57 Oral involvement in hand, foot and mouth disease.

9 / **Childhood infestations**

Head lice (pediculosis capitis)

Aetiology   Common infestation (Fig. 58) in unhygienic or crowded conditions.

Clinical features   Severe pruritus, especially on the nape of neck and occiput. Lice may be present, but nits (eggs) on hair shafts are diagnostic. Excoriations are common. Impetiginous secondary infection can occur. Exudation may cause matting of hair.

Treatment   Removal of nits with a fine-toothed metal comb. 0.5% malathion or 0.5% carbaryl solution is applied to hair after washing. Repeated treatments may be necessary. Contacts must also be treated.

Insect bites (papular urticaria)

Aetiology   Hypersensitivity reaction to insect bites, e.g. fleas, bedbugs, mites.

Clinical features   Urticated papules occur in groups (Figs 59 & 60) and may be seasonal. Bullae can occur, particularly on the legs. Pruritus may be intense. Episodes may be recurrent or persist for several months. Impetigo can be a complication.

Treatment   Symptomatic. Treat the source if possible (including pets). Systemic antihistamines and topical steroids may be useful.

See also Scabies (p. 89).

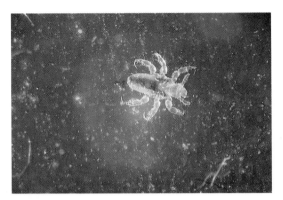

Fig. 58 Head louse.

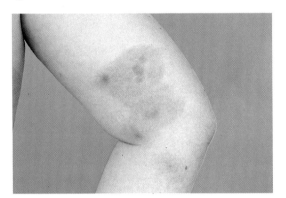

Fig. 59 Papular urticaria (bites).

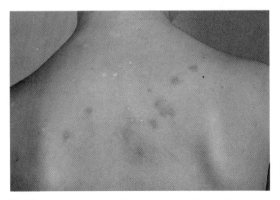

Fig. 60 Characteristic pattern of lesions as seen in insect bites.

10 / Childhood reactions

Henoch-Schönlein purpura (allergic vasculitis)

Aetiology

An immune complex hypersensitivity reaction to streptococcal infection.

Clinical features

Palpable (papular) purpura affects the lower legs, thighs and buttocks (Fig. 61); sometimes urticarial or necrotic. There may be arthralgia, abdominal pain, vomiting and bloody diarrhoea. Renal damage may lead to proliferative glomerulonephritis with nephritic or nephrotic syndromes. ESR and ASO titres may be raised. The urine should be checked regularly for protein, casts and haematuria.

Treatment

Bed-rest in the acute stage. Penicillin is administered for streptococcal infections; sometimes systemic steroids. Prognosis is generally good but depends on renal involvement.

Acute urticaria (hives; nettle rash)

Aetiology

Mast cell degranulation with histamine release due to drugs, foods, infections or infestations.

Clinical features

Increased incidence in atopics. Itchy weals arise suddenly, within minutes or hours (Figs 62 & 63). There may be associated angioedema and eosinophilia.

Treatment

Treat any underlying infestation or infection. Try elimination diets. Antihistamines can be helpful. Avoid aspirin.

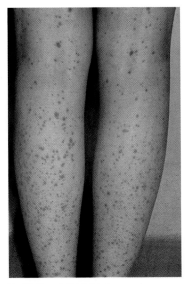

Fig. 61 Henoch-Schönlein type purpura.

Fig. 62 Urticarial weals.

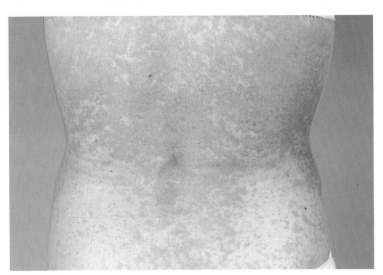

Fig. 63 Generalized urticaria.

11 / Acne vulgaris

Acne is an inflammatory disorder of the pilosebaceous follicles which occurs particularly at adolescence when sebaceous glands become active.

Aetiology

Several factors are of importance:
- genetic
- androgenic (and, to some degree, progesterogenic) stimulation
- abnormal sebum production
- colonization of pilosebaceous unit with *Propionibacterium acnes*
- obstruction of the sebaceous duct
- inflammation.

Clinical features

The characteristic lesion is the *comedone* (Fig. 64) which presents as a dark, follicular plug (blackhead), or a small papule (closed comedone). Secondary inflammation causes papules and pustules which may affect the face, chest, back and shoulders (Fig. 65). Pre-menstrual flares are common in women. Deeper *nodulocystic acne* produces severe scarring (Fig. 66) and occurs more commonly in men, as does *acne conglobata* (Fig. 67, p. 44), an uncommon, severe, recalcitrant form of acne. There are multiple 'paired' comedones with connecting sinuses, on the back, chest, neck and face. Large (conglobate) cysts may develop, and there is often scarring or acne-keloid formation (Figs 68 & 69, p. 44).

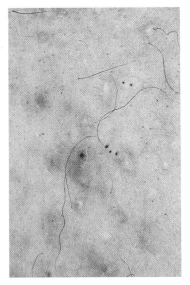

Fig. 64 Paired comedones as seen in acne conglobata.

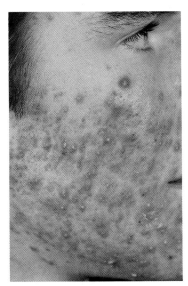

Fig. 65 Superficial inflammatory acne.

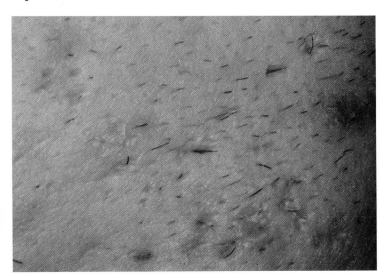

Fig. 66 Post acne ('ice-pick') scarring.

Management

Topical therapy

Keratolytics: beneficial for superficial inflammatory acne.

Benzoyl peroxide: both an antibacterial and a drying/peeling action.

Retinoic acid: useful for comedonal acne, although it may have an irritant effect. Intermittent use of the cream formulation is recommended initially.

Topical antibiotics: such as erythromycin, clindamycin or tetracycline in a propylene glycol and spirit base are of benefit in superficial inflammatory acne.

Ultraviolet B light and natural sunlight: often beneficial and produce erythema and slight peeling. Intralesional half-strength steroid is sometimes useful for inflammatory nodulocystic lesions.

Systemic therapy

Oral antibiotics: oxytetracycline or erythromycin 500 mg b.d. produce improvement in about 70% of patients. For tetracycline, it is important that *therapy* is taken with water and away from food. For maintenance therapy, antibiotics may be given at lower dose, but they will need to be continued for some months/years.

Oral contraceptives: containing higher levels of oestrogen doses, such as Dianette, may be helpful.

Oral retinoids (13 cis retinoic acid): can produce a dramatic improvement in severe nodulocystic acne. Teratogenic side-effects limit its use in women and the treatment is at present only available in hospital.

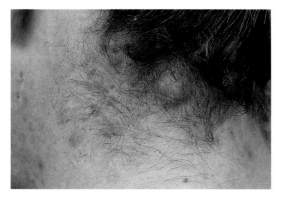

Fig. 67 Acne conglobata of neck.

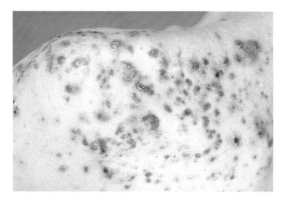

Fig. 68 Severe nodulocystic acne.

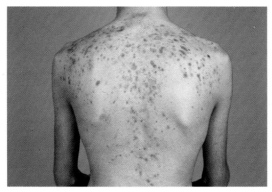

Fig. 69 Post-acne scarring.

12 / **Psoriasis**

Aetiology   Psoriasis affects approximately 2% of the population. Genetic factors are important: 40% of patients have a positive family history. There is a rapid epidermal transit time with increased epidermal cell production.

Clinical features   ***Plaque psoriasis:*** characterized by well-demarcated, erythematous areas covered with thick, silvery scales (Fig. 70). Pinpoint capillary bleeding occurs when scales are removed. Symmetrical plaques commonly affect extensor surfaces, especially the elbows and knees. The condition frequently affects the scalp and sacrum (Fig. 72), but patches may occur anywhere on the body, and at site of trauma (Koebner phenomenon) (Fig. 71).

Guttate (and exanthematic) psoriasis: (Figs 73, 74 & 75, p. 48) commoner in the young and often precipitated by a streptococcal sore throat. Multiple 'rain-drop' lesions occur suddenly on trunk and limbs. The condition may resolve spontaneously, or individual spots may enlarge and turn to plaque psoriasis.

Pustular psoriasis: rare generalized form which can be fatal. Patients are often erythrodermic with sheets of sterile pustules (Fig. 76, p. 48) and associated fever, malaise and leukocytosis.

Flexural psoriasis: the affected psoriatic skin loses its characteristic silvery scale, but the well-demarcated erythematous areas (Fig. 77, p. 50) remain and may mimic intertrigo, candidiasis and tinea.

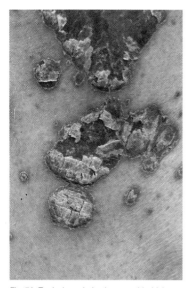

Fig. 70 Typical psoriatic plaques with thick silvery scales.

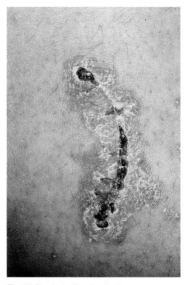

Fig. 71 Psoriasis showing Koebner phenomenon.

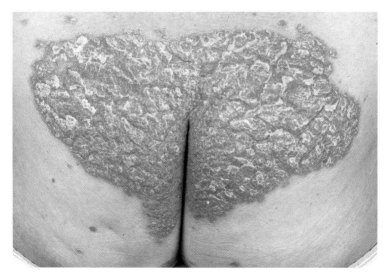

Fig. 72 Typical psoriatic plaque on sacrum.

Clinical features
(cont)

Erythrodermic psoriasis: when psoriasis involves the whole body the resulting erythroderma may be difficult to differentiate from other types of erythrodermic exfoliative dermatoses (Fig. 78, p. 50). Such patients lose their ability to control body temperature and fluid balance, and risk both infection and cardiac and renal failure.

Persistent palmoplantar pustulosis: this is often regarded as a localized form of psoriasis of the hands and feet, but frequently occurs without evidence of psoriasis elsewhere. Localized patches of erythema and scaling occur on the palms and soles (Fig. 79, p. 50) with scattered, sterile, yellow-brown pustules. The condition is very resistant to treatment.

Scalp psoriasis: multiple discrete plaques or involvement of the entire scalp and/or ears and scalp margins. Plaques are frequently thick, particularly at the occiput, but alopecia is uncommon (p. 151).

Nail psoriasis: the nails are commonly affected by several abnormalities in psoriasis, including pitting, onycholysis, subungual hyperkeratosis, salmon patch (p. 147).

Psoriatic arthropathy: commonly affects the terminal interphalangeal joints and sacroiliac joints, but both large and small joints may be involved. A severe destructive form of arthritis known as 'arthritis mutilans' is occasionally seen.

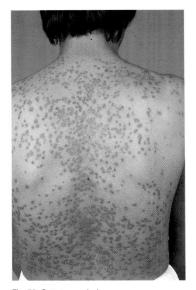

Fig. 73 Guttate psoriasis.

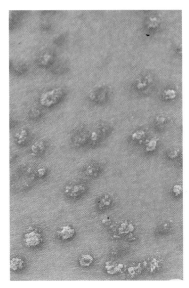

Fig. 74 Guttate psoriasis: raindrop lesions.

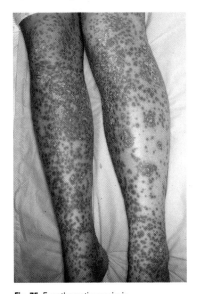

Fig. 75 Exanthematic psoriasis.

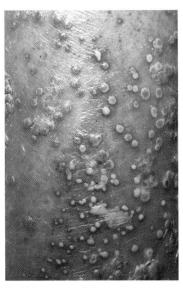

Fig. 76 Pustular psoriasis.

Treatment

Topical steroids: effective, but continued use may lead to lessening of effect and some destabilization of ordinary plaque psoriasis. These are better employed (in a descending sequence of potency) in combination with another treatment modality, e.g. tar. This combines the rapid initial benefits and cosmetic acceptability of topical steroids (by day) with the slower but more long-lasting effects of a coal tar preparation (at night). Weaker steroid or steroid/antiseptic preparations remain very useful for intertriginous areas.

Tar: can be used either alone or combined with salicylic acid. Cleaner forms are now available.

Ultraviolet light (UVB): E_0-E_1 dose alone or combined with tar/tar baths. A newer treatment combining psoralen with UVA (PUVA) is even more successful at clearing extensive refractory psoriasis.

Dithranol: useful for plaque psoriasis in in-patients. It is diluted in Lassar's Paste, initially at 0.1%. Cleaner forms are now available for out-patient use at normal concentrations overnight or in high concentrations for just half-an-hour. It may be combined with tar baths and UVB.

Vitamin D_3 ointment (calcipitriol): a new topical treatment for psoriasis, with an efficacy equivalent to topical steroids.

Systemic therapy: cytotoxic drugs, e.g. methotrexate, etretinate, cyclosporin, etc. are treatments normally only initiated by dermatologists.

Scalp psoriasis regimens: keratolytics, tar shampoos, topical steroids as lotions/gels.

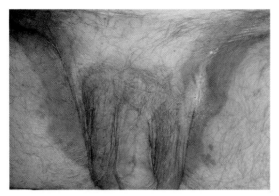

Fig. 77 Flexural psoriasis.

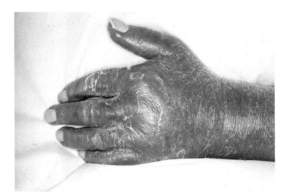

Fig. 78 Exfoliative/erythrodermic psoriasis.

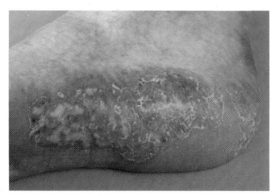

Fig. 79 Persistent palmoplantar pustulosis.

13 / Lichen planus

Aetiology The cause is unknown, although an autoimmune basis is likely.

Clinical features The characteristic skin lesions are small, itchy, shiny, flat-topped, violaceous papules (Fig. 80) with an overlying network of fine white lines (Wickham's striae) (Fig. 81). The eruption usually affects the wrists, forearms and trunk, lasting from 6 months to 2 years. The mouth (and genitalia) are also often affected with typical milky, 'lace-like' streaks or violaceous/atrophic patches. Scalp involvement may produce scarring alopecia, and permanent nail loss may occur if nail involvement is severe. Lesions occurring on the shins tend to coalesce and produce hypertrophic plaques (Fig. 82). Fading skin papules leave post-inflammatory hyperpigmentation. Lichen planus may also occur at sites of trauma (Fig. 83). This is known as the 'Koebner phenomenon' and is also seen in psoriasis and with certain viral infections such as molluscum contagiosum and plane warts.

Treatment Topical steroids and sedative antihistamines are helpful for symptomatic relief, although in mild cases no treatment may be required. Hypertrophic plaques can be treated with potent topical steroids or injected with intralesional steroids. There are also several proprietary steroid and anti-inflammatory agents that can be used for the mouth.

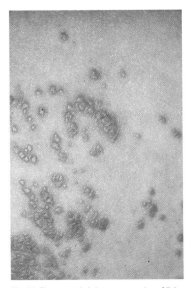

Fig. 80 Flat-topped violaceous papules of lichen planus.

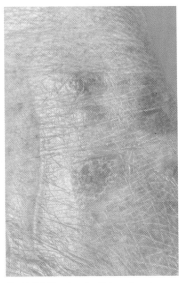

Fig. 81 Wickham's striae (lichen planus).

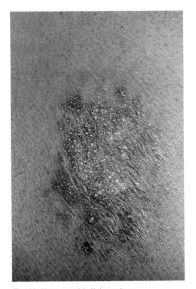

Fig. 82 Hypertrophic lichen planus.

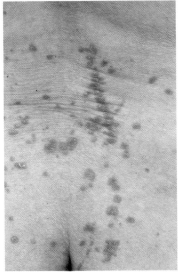

Fig. 83 Lichen planus (Koebner phenomenon).

14 / **Pityriasis rosea**

Pityriasis rosea is a common, self-limiting eruption which predominantly affects young adults.

Aetiology The cause is unknown; an infective agent has been suggested but not isolated.

Clinical features Characteristically, the initial lesion is a solitary oval, erythematous, scaly 'herald patch', often on the trunk (Fig. 84). Similar but smaller lesions appear after an interval of 1 or 2 weeks over the trunk, neck and upper arms in a symmetrical and generalized distribution. Individual lesions lie parallel to the ribs, creating a 'Christmas tree' pattern (Fig. 85). Pruritus is minimal, but occasionally there may be malaise and lymphadenopathy. The eruption usually fades within 4–6 weeks.

Management Usually no treatment is required. Mild topical steroids may hasten resolution or help the more 'eczematous' cases.

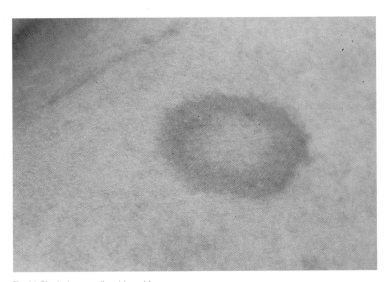

Fig. 84 Pityriasis rosea: 'herald patch'.

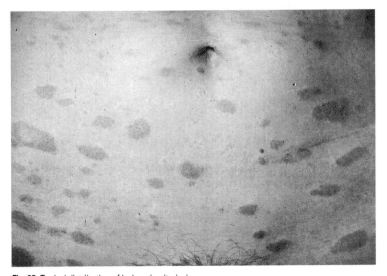

Fig. 85 Typical distribution of lesions in pityriasis rosea.

15 / **Pityriasis lichenoides**

Aetiology Unknown.

Clinical features Two forms exist:
- acute
- chronic.

Acute: adolescents are usually affected. Small, red papules occur on the trunk and limbs. The lesions become vesicular and then necrotic and ulcerate to produce pitted scars. Fever and systemic upset may occur. Mucous membranes may be involved. The eruption is often mistaken for chickenpox (Figs 86 & 87).

Chronic: small, reddish or orange-brown papules occur. Some may become purpuric whilst others develop a characteristic 'mica' scale. Lesions resolve slowly, leaving either a brown hyperpigmented or hypopigmented area. There is no systemic upset. The condition may grumble on for months or years (Figs 88 & 89).

Treatment None may be necessary. Ultraviolet light (UVB), PUVA and sunshine are all useful in the chronic form. Tar baths may be combined with both sun and UVB.

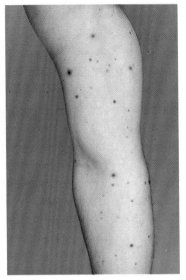

Fig. 86 Pityriasis lichenoides acuta.

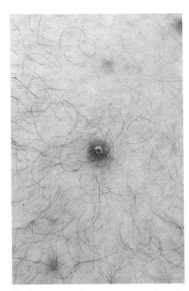

Fig. 87 Close-up of an early lesion of pityriasis lichenoides.

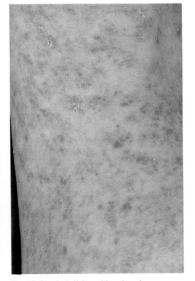

Fig. 88 Pityriasis lichenoides chronica.

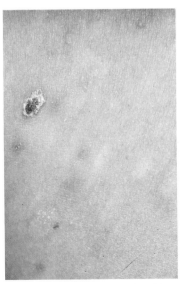

Fig. 89 Pityriasis lichenoides chronica with post-inflammatory hypopigmentation.

Chronic urticaria (hives, nettle-rash)

Aetiology An increase in vascular permeability/reactivity. Both immune (type I and III) and non-immune (pharmacological) mechanisms may play a part. Histamine is the most common mediator. Frequent precipitating factors include:

- drugs, e.g. aspirin, penicillin
- food additives, e.g. tartrazine (E102)
- fungal/yeast infections, e.g. thrush
- parasites, e.g. intestinal worms
- other infections
- disorders of the immune system, e.g. SLE, complement deficiency
- stress.

In many cases no obvious cause is found.

Clinical features Transient raised weals varying from a few mm to several cm in size (Figs 90 & 91). Limbs and trunk are particularly affected but lesions may occur anywhere. Weals are extremely itchy, last from 4–24 hours and fade completely. Pressure sites are commonly affected and most patients are also dermographic (Fig. 92). There may be associated angioedema. Rarely, there is overlap with urticarial vasculitis.

Treatment Avoid aspirin and any other drugs that may have been implicated. Treat any underlying bacterial, fungal or parasitic infection. Elimination diets (especially a dye and preservative-free diet) may help. Antihistamines give relief; severely affected patients may require systemic steroids.

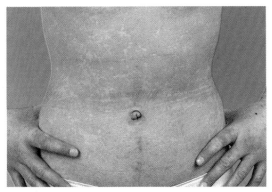

Fig. 90 Giant urticaria.

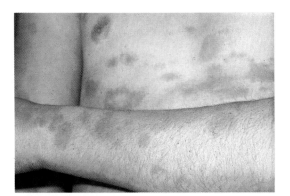

Fig. 91 Urticarial weals.

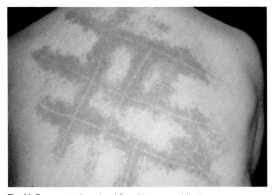

Fig. 92 Exaggerated weal and flare (dermographism).

Angioedema

Aetiology

Hereditary angioedema is an autosomal dominant condition due to C1 esterase inhibitor deficiency in the complement cascade. Angioedema may also occur as part of the symptom complex in both acute and chronic urticaria. Nuts and fish/shellfish are the most common dietary allergic causes.

Clinical features

Angioedema produces swelling of the lips (Figs 93 & 94), periorbital area (Fig. 95), neck and joints. The larynx may be affected and such involvement can be fatal. Gut involvement may produce abdominal pains. Urticaria is not normally a feature of true hereditary angioedema but the latter may occur in cases of ordinary urticaria.

Treatment

Anyone who suffers recurrent attacks of angioedema or in whom there is a family history of angioedema should be positively screened for C1 esterase inhibitor deficiency. Specific drugs such as stanozolol, tranexamic acid and danazol are the only effective prophylactic agents for hereditary angioedema. Acute episodes require injection of C1 esterase inhibitor or infusion of fresh frozen plasma. Angioedema associated with ordinary urticaria may be treated with antihistamines and/or steroids. Severe attacks should be treated as for anaphylaxis, with 0.5 ml 1/1 000 adrenalin by subcutaneous injection.

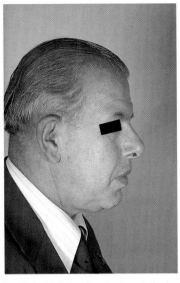

Fig. 93 Aspirin-induced angioedema (before).

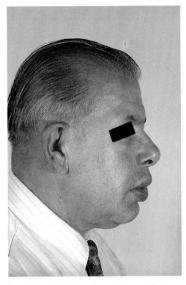

Fig. 94 Aspirin-induced angioedema (after).

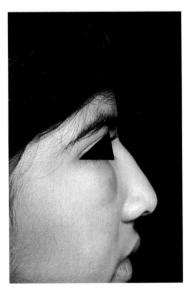

Fig. 95 Periorbital swelling (recurrent angioedema).

17 / Systemic reaction patterns

Erythema multiforme

Aetiology A localized form of vasculitis. Attacks may be triggered by drugs and viral infections (especially herpes simplex and *Mycoplasma*).

Clinical features The eruption can occur at any age. There may be a prodromal illness. Initial lesions are dull, red, flat maculopapules spreading centrifugally, the centre becoming cyanotic, purpuric or even bullous or necrotic (Fig. 96). The characteristic target or iris lesions (Fig. 97) symmetrically involve the periphery, e.g. palms, dorsae of hands, feet, knees, elbows and forearms. Mucous membranes may be affected. A severe bullous form of erythema multiforme, Stevens-Johnson syndrome, with particular involvement of mucous membranes, can occur (Fig. 98). There is associated pyrexia and malaise, with oral, ocular and genital lesions. This form carries a significant morbidity and mortality.

Treatment Usually symptomatic. Steroids may reduce the severity of attacks. The underlying cause should be removed or treated, where possible. Patients with severe recurrent erythema multiforme caused by herpes simplex may require treatment with continuous prophylactic acyclovir or by regular bi-monthly injections of gamma-globulin.

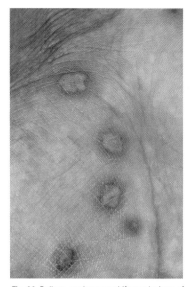

Fig. 96 Bullous erythema multiforme lesions of palm.

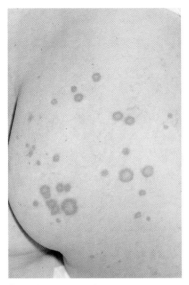

Fig. 97 Erythema multiforme: typical target or iris lesions.

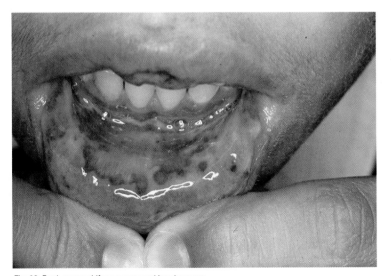

Fig. 98 Erythema multiforme: mucosal involvement.

Erythema nodosum

Aetiology   A common vasculitic reaction of larger subcutaneous vessels, due to a variety of provoking agents.
- Sarcoidosis.
- Infections.
  - streptococcus
  - tuberculosis
  - infectious mononucleosis
  - viral
  - chlamydia.
- Drugs
  - sulphonamides
  - oral contraceptives
  - salicylates
  - bromides/iodides
  - gold salts.
- Inflammatory bowel disease.

Clinical features   There may be a prodromal illness. Erythematous, tender, nodules appear on shins (Fig. 99) and occasionally thighs and forearms. There is associated pyrexia, malaise, oedema and aching of legs. The colour changes from bright red to purple to leave a brownish 'bruise'. Lesions occur in crops and recurrences may occur. Most attacks settle within 2–12 weeks.

Treatment   Bed-rest, anti-inflammatory analgesics and support stockings or bandages. Systemic steroids may be required for severe cases.

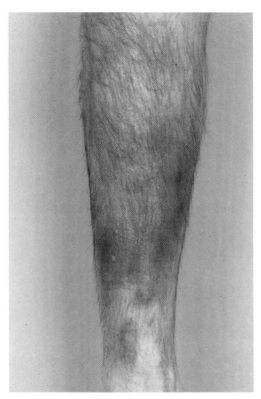

Fig. 99 Erythema nodosum.

Vasculitis

Aetiology Immune complex deposition in blood vessels. Drugs, infections, ingested allergens and autoantigens have all been implicated.

Clinical features Classically, the lower legs are affected, but the arms and trunk can also be involved (Fig. 100). Urticaria, toxic erythema and palpable purpura may progress to necrotic or bullous lesions (Fig. 101) with crusting and ulceration. Possible associated systemic vasculitis with renal, gastrointestinal and respiratory involvement and arthritis.

Treatment Investigation of the underlying cause; bed-rest. Systemic steroids may be required.

Capillaritis

Aetiology Capillary leakage/vasculitis (Fig. 102). Most causes are cryptogenic, e.g. Schamberg's capillaritis, but some drugs produce a similar eruption. Stasis factors are also important.

Clinical features The idiopathic type usually affects the lower legs of young men. Discrete areas of asymptomatic red-brown, petechial or punctate purpura—become hyperpigmented.

Treatment Support stockings may help.

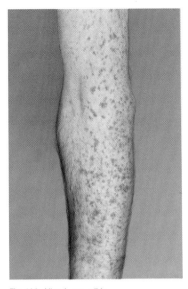

Fig. 100 Allergic vasculitis.

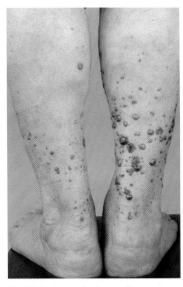

Fig. 101 Leukocytoclastic vasculitis.

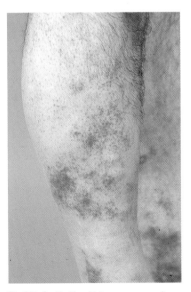

Fig. 102 Capillaritis with 'cayenne pepper' pigmentation.

18 / Rosacea

Aetiology	Unknown. Increased lability and reactivity of the facial vasculature.
Clinical features	Initially, transient flushing but later a persistent and diffuse facial erythema with inflamed papules and pustules (acne rosacea) (Fig. 103) and telangiectasia. It chiefly involves glabella, cheeks, nose and chin. Lymphoedema, conjunctival suffusion, conjunctivitis, blepharitis and (rarely) keratitis are seen. It may be exacerbated by sun, heat, alcohol and hot/spicy foods. It is more common in women, especially those with fair or celtic skin. *Rhinophyma* (Fig. 104) is a variant seen mainly in men in which there is enlargement of the nose due to hypertrophy of sebaceous glands.
Treatment	Avoid precipitating factors. Oral oxytetracycline (papules and pustules) and oral clonidine (flushing). Topical 1% metronidazole is also effective. Rhinophyma usually requires plastic surgery. Low-dose antibiotics needed for months/years. Topical steroids are contraindicated.

Perioral dermatitis

Aetiology	Unknown. It may develop from paraoral acne or paranasal seborrhoeic dermatitis. Prior use of a potent topical steroid is usually a factor.
Clinical features	Papulopustular eruption on a scaly, erythematous background around the mouth, nose and nasolabial folds. It is more frequent in women (Fig. 105).
Treatment	Systemic oxytetracycline (a reducing 4–6 week course), and 1% hydrocortisone cream to reduce 'rebound' when potent steroids withdrawn.

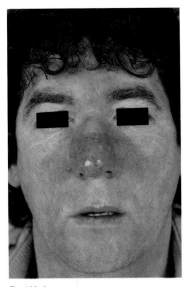

Fig. 103 Acne rosacea.

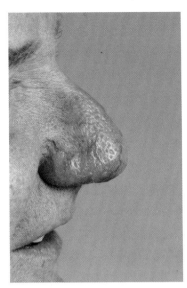

Fig. 104 Rhinophyma.

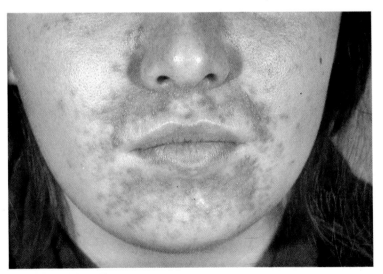

Fig. 105 Perioral dermatitis.

19 / Physical urticarias

Dermographism

Clinical features   Light pressure produces a weal and flare formation with itching at the site of trauma within 5 min (Fig. 106). It may be associated with chronic urticaria, and is asymptomatic in around 5% of normal population.

Treatment   None may be required, or antihistamines.

Cholinergic urticaria

Clinical features   Common, predominantly affecting young adults and involving mainly trunk and limbs. Extremely itchy, micropapular, urticarial weals occur in response to exercise, emotion or heat (Fig. 107).

Treatment   Antihistamines and anticholinergics may be helpful. It tends to resolve spontaneously.

Pressure urticaria

Clinical features   Rare; may be a component of ordinary chronic urticaria. Continued pressure produces painful swollen, indurated urticarial areas after several hours (Fig. 108). It may persist for 1–2 days.

Treatment   Cyproheptadine or other antihistamines can be tried, but the response is often disappointing. Oral steroids may be required.

Other physical urticarias

Clinical features   May be initiated by cold, heat, ultraviolet light, vibration and contact with water. Sometimes itching is the only feature.

Treatment   Antihistamines; avoidance of trigger factors; sunblocks for those reacting to light; advice on the dangers of swimming for those with cold urticaria.

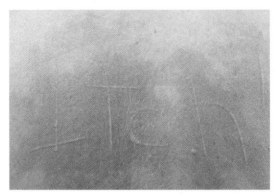

Fig. 106 Dermographism.

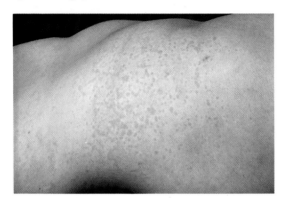

Fig. 107 Cholinergic urticaria.

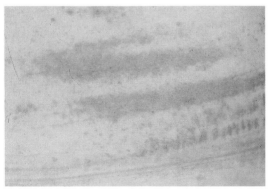

Fig. 108 Pressure urticaria.

20 / **Photosensitive eruptions**

Polymorphic light eruption (PMLE)

Clinical features Relatively common; usually affects young women, although it may occur at any age. Itchy papules or papulovesicles, erythema and urticated plaques develop within hours, mainly at sites recently exposed to sun (Fig. 109). Starts in spring/early summer and declines thereafter. Tends to recur over many years. Sometimes associated with solar urticaria.

Treatment Clothing and high protection broad-spectrum sunscreens or sunblocks. Topical steroids and oral antihistamines. Tolerance can be induced. PUVA or UVB therapy can be given prophylactically to those severely affected. Mepacrine, hydroxychloroquine or systemic steroids are sometimes required for severe cases.

Hutchinson's summer prurigo

Clinical features Affects young children. There may be a family history. Itchy, erythematous, often excoriated papules on cheeks (Fig. 110), nose and dorsum of hands.

Treatment Symptomatic. Sunscreens partially helpful.

Juvenile spring eruption

Clinical features Uncommon condition seen in boys more than girls. Erythema and pruritus of the ears is followed by grouped papules and vesicles. Cold may be a contributory factor. No treatment.

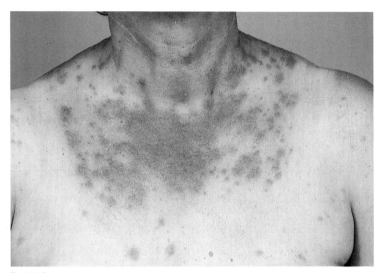

Fig. 109 Polymorphic light eruption.

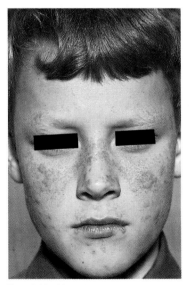

Fig. 110 Hutchinson's summer prurigo.

Photosensitive eczema/actinic reticuloid

Aetiology
- Secondary to some eczemas—childhood atopic; seborrhoeic dermatitis in older men; volatile contact dermatitis, e.g. to Compositae.
- Topically applied chemicals—tar, creosote.
- Systemic drugs—thiazides, phenothiazines.

Clinical features Mainly seen in the summer. Sensitivity is usually confined to short-wave UVL (UVB)/exposed areas, but in actinic reticuloid may extend to include UVA and visible light, and may be year-long and generalized. Drug-induced photosensitivity is normally due to long-wave UVL (UVA) (Figs 111 & 112).

Treatment Elimination of drug/easily avoided environmental causes. In constitutional eczema or those sensitized to a ubiquitous allergen, symptomatic treatment with topical steroids and broad-spectrum sunscreens. In severe cases, systemic steroids and azathioprine.

Solar urticaria

Aetiology Unknown; abnormal reactivity to UVL.

Clinical features Rare. There is development of severely pruritic, erythematous weals within a few minutes of sun exposure which resolve within about 1 h of sun avoidance. Erythropoietic protoporphyria must be excluded.

Treatment Sun avoidance; antihistamines no help.

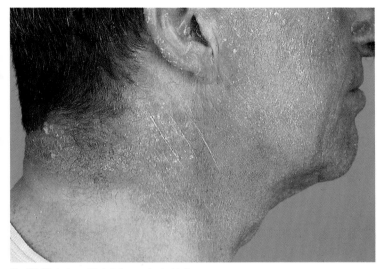

Fig. 111 Photodermatitis/relative sparing behind ear.

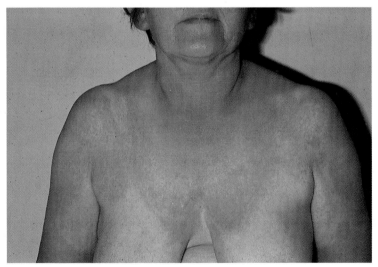

Fig. 112 Drug-induced photosensitivity.

Discoid lupus erythematosus

Aetiology   Autoimmune disorder.

Clinical features   Symmetrical, well-defined plaques of erythema with scaling, atrophy and follicular plugging (Fig. 113). It mainly affects light-exposed areas such as face, neck, scalp, ears, upper chest, back and backs of hands (Figs 114 & 115), and is frequently exacerbated by sunlight. Scalp involvement may produce scarring alopecia (Fig. 116). Rarely, there may also be associated systemic symptoms of lupus erythematosus.

Treatment   Avoidance of sunlight. Sunscreens and topical steroids are helpful. Mepacrine, hydrochloroquine or systemic steroids may be required.

Skin disorders usually aggravated by sunlight

These include polymorphic light eruption and other photodermatoses, lupus erythematosus, porphyrias, rosacea, herpes simplex, erythema multiforme and benign lymphocytic infiltrations.

Skin disorders usually helped by sunlight

These include psoriasis, acne vulgaris, pityriasis lichenoides, 'parapsoriasis' and mycosis fungoides.

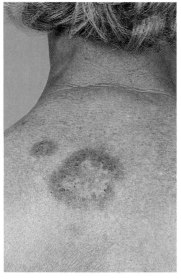

Fig. 113 Discoid lupus erythematosus.

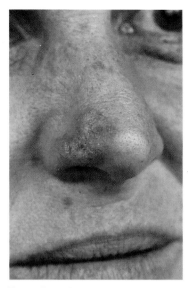

Fig. 114 Well-defined plaque of DLE on nose with follicular plugging/scarring.

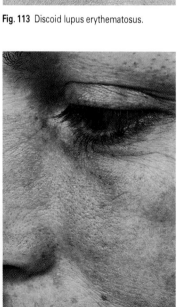

Fig. 115 Classical 'butterfly' distribution of DLE.

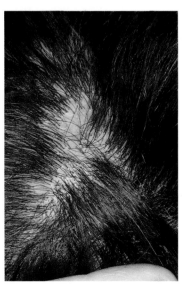

Fig. 116 Scarring alopecia.

21 / **Drug reactions/Eruptions**

The wide availability and use of drugs makes a drug history extremely important.

Aetiology   Hypersensitivity reactions can occur where the drug or drug metabolite acts as an antigen. However, many eruptions remain idiosyncratic.

Clinical features   Urticarial (p. 39), eczematous, bullous and lichenoid reactions may be seen. Specific eruption patterns include the following.

Morbilliform: common maculopapular pattern of drug eruption which mimics viral exanthems. A good example of this is the ampicillin rash in patients with glandular fever. Other antibiotics and phenothiazines may give a similar reaction pattern (Fig. 117).

Vasculitis (Fig. 118): produced by many drugs, including sulphonamides (see p. 65).

Erythema multiforme/Stevens-Johnson syndrome: typical target lesions may be caused by barbiturates, phenytoin, gold, phenylbutazone and sulphonamides. Severe cases can progress to Stevens-Johnson syndrome with severe mucosal involvement (Fig. 119).

Purpuric: drugs can produce purpura (Fig. 120, p. 80) by direct capillary damage or via thrombocytopenia, e.g. gold salts, quinine, quinidine, thiazides and benzodiazepines.

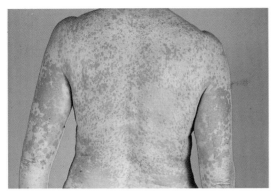

Fig. 117 Morbilliform 'ampicillin'-type rash.

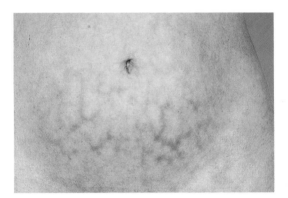

Fig. 118 Livedo vasculitis.

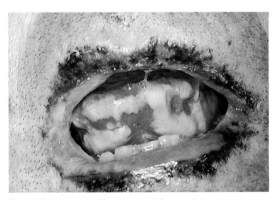

Fig. 119 Severe mucosal involvement in Stevens-Johnson syndrome.

Clinical features   **Toxic epidermal necrolysis:** large areas of epidermis are lost, leaving extensive, denuded areas of skin (p. 29). Fluid loss, electrolyte imbalance and secondary infection are frequent complications. The condition has a significant mortality and may be caused by potent drugs including barbiturates, sulphonamides, hydantoin, phenylbutazone and other non-steroidal anti-inflammatories.

Fixed drug eruption: these lesions are characteristically well demarcated and dusky red, often with central blistering (Fig. 121) and subsequent post-inflammatory pigmentation. The eruption occurs at the same sites each time the responsible drug is taken. Laxatives containing phenol-phthalein, barbiturates and sulphonamides are common offenders.

Photosensitivity: phototoxic reactions can occur with drugs which would not usually produce a skin eruption without sun exposure (p. 71). The distribution is typical, being confined to exposed areas, e.g. face, arms and 'V' of neck. Shaded areas such as those under the chin and ears are often spared. Photoallergic reactions can also occur. Thiazides, sulphonamides, chlorpromazine, tetracyclines and nalidixic acid may all be responsible (Fig. 122). Post-inflammatory pigmentation may occur with some drugs, especially amiodarone (Fig. 123).

Treatment   Withdrawal of offending drug; systemic steroids occasionally.

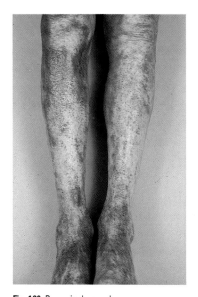

Fig. 120 Purpuric drug rash.

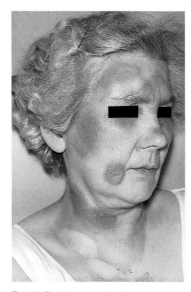

Fig. 121 Fixed drug eruption due to barbiturates, sulphonamides, etc.

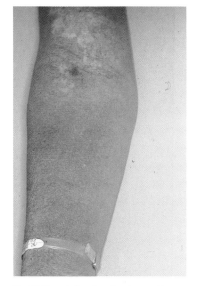

Fig. 122 Drug-induced erythroderma with islands of normal skin.

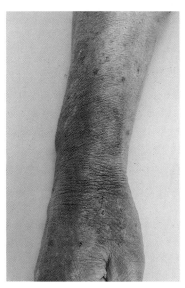

Fig. 123 Amiodarone pigmentation.

Dermatitis herpetiformis

Aetiology An autoimmune disease associated with gluten enteropathy and IgA in the skin.

Clinical features Groups of small blisters or papulovesicles on an urticated background involving elbows, knees, buttocks, scalp and scapular areas. Intensely itchy excoriations rather than blisters are usually seen (Figs 124 & 125).

Treatment Can be controlled by dapsone. A strict gluten-free diet is necessary.

Pemphigus

Aetiology Autoimmune disease directed against epidermal cells and intraepidermal cement.

Clinical features A disease of the middle-aged, especially Jews. Widespread, erythematous erosions (or true blisters) can occur on any area of the body (Fig. 126). Firm pressure on the surrounding skin will produce a sore. Mucous membranes are also involved. It tends to be fatal if left untreated.

Treatment High doses of systemic steroids initially; azathioprine as a steroid-sparing agent.

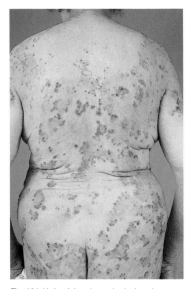

Fig. 124 Urticarial and annular lesions in dermatitis herpetiformis.

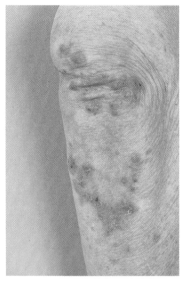

Fig. 125 The elbows are a characteristic site of involvement in dermatitis herpetiformis.

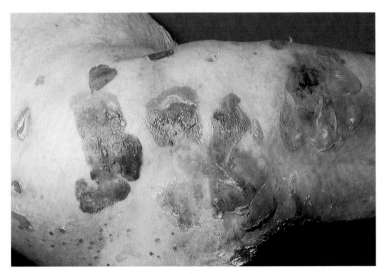

Fig. 126 Flaccid blisters and erosions (pemphigus).

Pemphigoid

Aetiology Autoimmune disease directed against the basement membrane of the skin.

Clinical features A disease of the elderly. An urticated eruption develops initially (often on the limbs—Fig. 127) blisters usually appearing within a few days. Irritation can be intense. Blisters are large, thick-walled, tense and do not rupture easily (Fig. 128). Disease soon becomes widespread and symmetrical. Mucosal involvement is relatively uncommon.

Treatment High doses of systemic steroids initially; lower maintenance dose for several months. Azathioprine may be used as a steroid-sparing agent. Dapsone and potent topical steroids may be effective for mild or localized disease.

Cicatricial (mucosal) pemphigoid

Aetiology Autoimmune disease closely related to pemphigoid.

Clinical features A disease of the elderly. Blisters rupture to produce superficial erosions which heal with scarring. The mucous membrane of the mouth and conjunctivae are most frequently affected (Fig. 129), but the nose, throat, genitalia, anus and oesophagus can be involved. Scarring causes adhesions between conjunctival surfaces and scarring alopecia on the scalp.

Treatment Systemic steroids may be required. Occular involvement must be treated by an ophthalmologist.

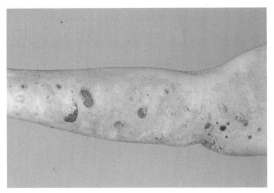

Fig. 127 Urticated and bullous lesions of pemphigoid.

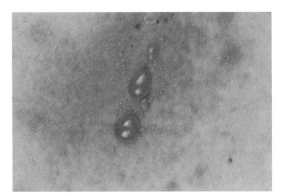

Fig. 128 Tense blisters in bullous pemphigoid.

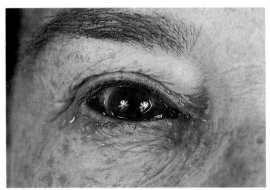

Fig. 129 Mucosal involvement in case of cicatricial pemphigoid.

23 / Bacterial infections

Staphylococcus aureus

Clinical features

Boils/furuncles: staphylococcal hair follicle abcesses—painful, red papules becoming pustular to heal with scarring. Atopy, diabetes and poor hygiene predispose. Patients may carry *Staph. aureus* in nose or perineum between attacks.

Folliculitis (Fig. 130): superficial staphylococcal infection of hair follicles, with small discrete pustules of beard, neck, scalp, buttocks and limbs.

Treatment

Antibiotics. Recurrent infections require swabs and appropriate antibiotics. Treat carriers (including family members) with antibiotic nasal cream and antiseptic baths/powder.

Streptococcus pyogenes

Clinical features

Erysipelas: due to superficial infection with streptococci—tender, red and oedematous skin with a sharply demarcated, indurated edge.

Cellulitis (Fig. 131): a deeper streptococcal infection with an ill-defined edge. It commonly involves face and legs, and there may be associated lymphangitis, fever/rigors and systemic toxicity. Diabetes, incompetent lymphatics and poor health predispose.

Treatment

Intramuscular penicillin. A penicillinase-resistant antibiotic (e.g. flucloxacillin) may need to be added for combined strep./staph. infections. Erythromycin can be used for those allergic to penicillin.

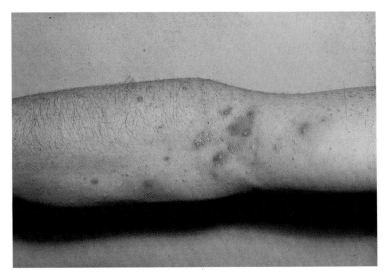

Fig. 130 Folliculitis.

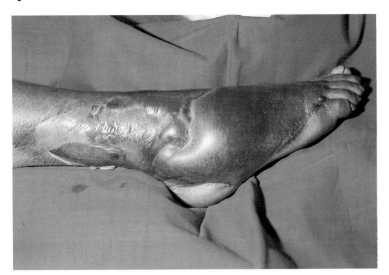

Fig. 131 Bullous cellulitis.

24 / Herpes infection

Herpes simplex

Aetiology Type I normally causes herpes labialis, and type II causes genital infections.

Clinical features **Primary herpes simplex** (Fig. 132) mainly occurs in children as stomatitis, fever and lymphadenopathy. Recurrent infections are characterized by *herpes labialis* ('cold sore') with small, closely grouped vesicles on an erythematous base. *Eczema herpeticum* occurs in patients with atopic eczema and in the immunosuppressed.

Treatment Use topical antiseptics, idoxuridine, or acyclovir for cold sores, and oral acyclovir for severe/generalized herpes.

Herpes zoster

Aetiology Varicella-zoster virus (dormant in dorsal root ganglion after childhood chickenpox).

Clinical features Pain in the affected dermatome. After 1–3 days, there are clustered, red papules which become vesicular then pustular (Fig. 133). There may be fever, malaise and lymphadenopathy. Pain may persist for months. Involvement of ophthalmic division of trigeminal nerve may cause keratitis/blindness. Dissemination occurs in the immunosuppressed.

Treatment Treat as for herpes simplex. For post-herpetic neuralgia, use analgesics, carbamazepine, tricyclic antidepressants (or oral steroids, if given early).

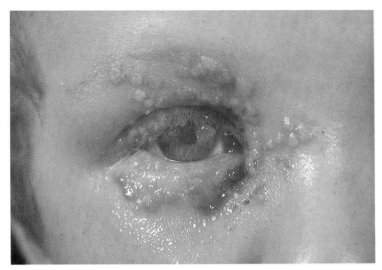

Fig. 132 Herpes simplex. A pustular and crusted eruption with fever, malaise and prostration.

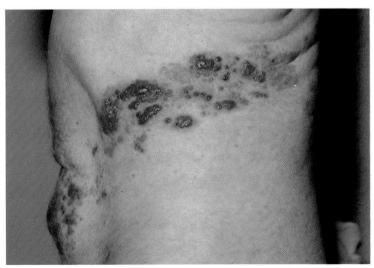

Fig. 133 Typical dermatomal distribution of herpes zoster.

25 / **Infestations**

Scabies

Aetiology
Sarcoptes scabiei var. *hominis*. Eggs are laid in epidermal burrows by the female acarus (mite). Overcrowding and sexual promiscuity predispose.

Clinical features
Pruritus is severe, intractable and worse at night, commencing about 2 weeks after the primary infection when the patient has developed hypersensitivity to the mite. Characteristic burrows (Fig. 134) are seen in finger webs and on flexor aspects of wrists, with characteristic papules on penis (Fig. 135), buttocks and around areolae. Vesicles may occur, but excoriations are more common (Fig. 136). Impetigo may coexist. Indurated, inflammatory nodules are sometimes seen on the scrotum and elsewhere. Lesions do not affect the head, except in infants, who often also have lesions around the umbilicus. The acarus can be demonstrated by scraping a burrow and examining the contents in 20% KOH under a microscope.

Treatment
Topical malathion 0.5%, benzyl benzoate BP, 1% gamma benzene hexachloride, applied at night and repeated if necessary one week later. Children are probably best treated with aqueous malathion lotion. Crotamiton cream or lotion can be used later to treat pruritus and/or to prevent recurrence. Treatment should be combined with a change of contact clothing/bedding. All close contacts and all members of the household must be treated whether clinically affected or not.

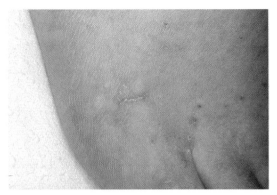

Fig. 134 Characteristic burrow of scabies.

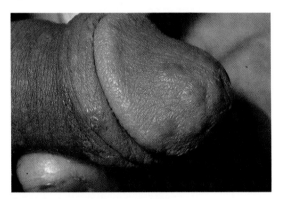

Fig. 135 Persistent penile papules (scabies).

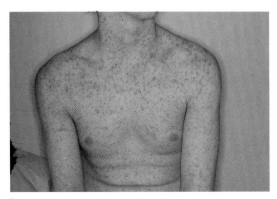

Fig. 136 Widespread pruritis rash of scabies.

Lice

Aetiology Lice are translucent, wingless insects. Poor hygiene and crowded conditions predispose.

Clinical features **Head louse:** (p. 37).

Body louse: asymptomatic pinpoint red macules. Pruritus, excoriations, papular urticaria and secondary infection follow, with hyperpigmentation in chronic cases (Fig. 137). Lice and eggs are found in the seams of clothing.

Pubic louse: often transmitted by sexual contact. There is intense pruritus of the pubic region. The eggs (nits) appear as grains of sand attached to the hair shafts.

Treatment Remove nits with a fine-toothed metal comb. Treat with 0.5% carbaryl/0.5% malathion lotions. Contacts must also be treated. A thorough disinfection of clothing is necessary.

Larva migrans

Aetiology The larvae of various worms, e.g. *Ancylostoma braziliense, Strongyloides stercoralis.*

Clinical features The larvae penetrate the skin of feet, hands or buttocks. They migrate, producing intensely itchy, raised, red serpentine lines (Fig. 138).

Treatment Local application of 10% thiabendazole suspension or oral thiabendazole.

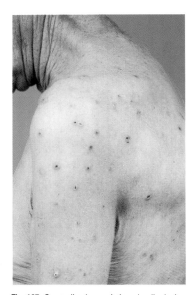

Fig. 137 Generalized excoriations (pediculosis corporis).

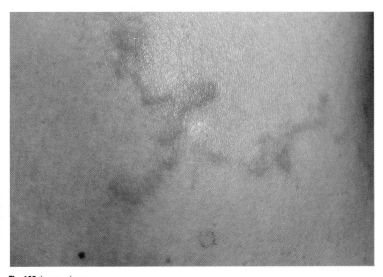

Fig. 138 Larva migrans.

26 / Fungal infections

Aetiology Ringworm (tinea) infections enzymatically digest keratin. Obtain scrapings for microscopy and culture before beginning treatment. Infections are classified as follows:

- Tinea pedis (athlete's foot) is due to *Trichophyton rubrum*, T. *interdigitale* and *Epidermophyton floccosum*. It is precipitated by communal showering, swimming pools and occlusive footwear.
- Tinea manuum is predominantly due to *T. rubrum*.
- Tinea cruris is caused by the same organisms as tinea pedis.
- Tinea corporis is caused by all types of ringworm.

Clinical features **Tinea pedis** (Figs 139 & 141): scaling, fissuring or irritation, especially between 4th and 5th toes. It may also be caused by bacteria, *Candida* or sweating, and may produce erythema, scaling and occasionally vesicles/pustules on sole of foot.

Tinea manuum (Fig. 140): characteristically unilateral with scaling of the palm. Exaggerated skin markings are also seen.

Tinea cruris: occurs predominantly in young men. There is well demarcated erythema and scaling in the groins with central clearing and an 'active' edge (Fig. 142, p. 96).

Tinea corporis: discoid, scaly areas which spread slowly with central clearing. The edge of the lesion may be vesicular (Fig. 143, p. 96).

Treatment Topical antifungal agents e.g. Whitfield's ointment or imidazole creams/lotion, Castellani's paint for interdigital maceration. Griseofulvin 500 mg daily (with food) for 4–5 weeks or one of the newer oral antifungals such as terbinafine or itraconazole may be necessary for *T. rubrum* or more extensive infections.

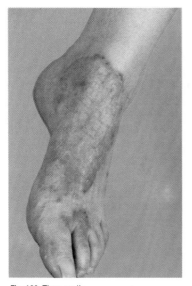

Fig. 139 Tinea pedis.

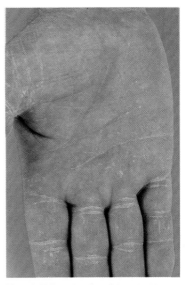

Fig. 140 Unilateral scaling of the palm (tinea manuum).

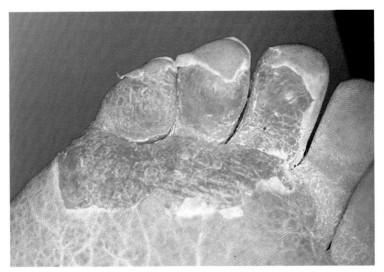

Fig. 141 Dermatophyte infection spreading out from the toes.

Tinea incognito

Aetiology Ringworm infection modified by topical (or systemic) steroids (Fig. 139, p. 94, and Fig. 144).

Clinical features The inflammatory response is suppressed by use of steroids. Itching and inflammation are reduced, the margins less distinct and scaling less apparent, yet slowly enlarging.

Treatment Topical imidazole and oral griseofulvin or other systemic agent. There may be some increase in inflammation on stopping the steroid.

Majocchi's ringworm granuloma

Aetiology A foreign body granulomatous reaction due to folliculitis from *Trichophyton rubrum* (Fig. 144).

Clinical features Predominantly in adults; an erythematous, scaly plaque on a limb studded with follicular pustules. The plaque is unilateral, but may spread to involve the whole limb.

Treatment Oral griseofulvin 500 mg daily or other systemic antifungal for 4–6 weeks.

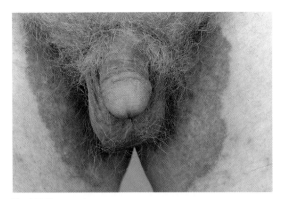

Fig. 142 Tinea cruris.

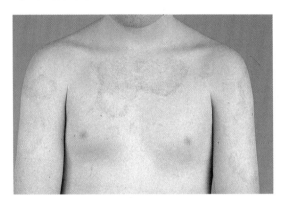

Fig. 143 Tinea corporis.

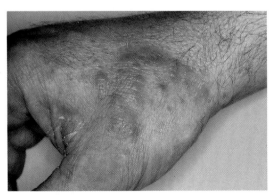

Fig. 144 Majocchi's granuloma.

27 / Fungal/Yeast/Bacterial infections

Pityriasis versicolor (tinea versicolor)

Aetiology *Pityrosporum orbiculare*. The condition is common in hot, humid environments. The condition presents as hyperpigmented or hypopigmented macules with fine superficial scales (Figs 145 & 146), mostly on the trunk or upper limbs and often more conspicuous following sunbathing.

Treatment Selenium sulphide or ketoconazole shampoos, and topical imidazole creams. Oral itraconazole may be used in resistant cases. It may take several months for normal skin colour to return, and the condition tends to relapse.

Candidiasis

Aetiology *Candida albicans*; moisture, warmth, occlusion, antibiotics, steroid treatment, pregnancy and immunosuppression all predispose.

Clinical features Erythema with scaling (Fig. 147) and papular or pustular satellite lesions at and beyond a well defined irregular edge, affecting skin folds, especially in obese patients (intertrigo). It may be itchy or sore. (See also napkin candidiasis on page 15).

Treatment Nystatin or imidazole creams; eradication of gut and vaginal yeast carriage; oral fluconasole in resistant cases.

Erythrasma

Aetiology Diphtheroid *Corynebacterium minutissimum*.

Clinical features Well demarcated brownish erythema in axillae, groins and toe webs with superficial scaling; fluoresces coral-pink under Wood's light.

Treatment Fucidin or imidazole cream; systemic erythromycin.

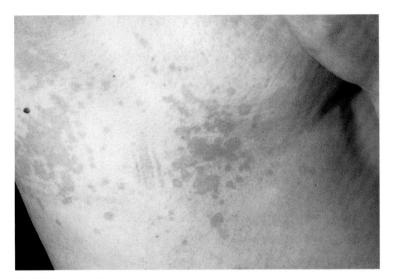

Fig. 145 Pityriasis versicolor.

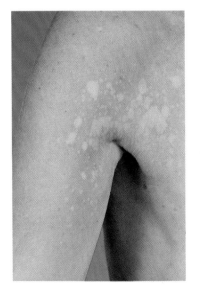

Fig. 146 Hypopigmented lesions of pityriasis versicolor.

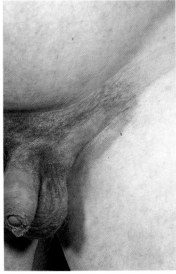

Fig. 147 Candidal intertrigo.

Seborrhoeic wart (basal cell papilloma)

Aetiology Often familial.

Clinical features Common in both sexes in middle life, usually on the trunk, increasing in number and size with age. It is characteristically yellow-brown/black and greasy with a rough craggy surface (Fig. 148).

Differential diagnosis Malignant melanoma; pigmented basal cell carcinoma.

Treatment Curettage (with application of superficial styptic); cryotherapy.

Skin tag (fibroepithelial polyp)

Aetiology Familial: obesity, pregnancy.

Clinical features Multiple, soft, round and peduncular with a narrow base (Fig. 149). These characteristically occur on the neck, axillae and groins.

Treatment 'Snip' and cautery; diathermy.

Solar lentigo ('senile'/actinic lentigo)

Aetiology Excessive exposure to sunlight.

Clinical features A brown macule—often multiple—occurring on light-exposed skin of fair-skinned individuals. (Fig. 150).

Differential diagnosis Lentigo maligna.

Treatment None. Cosmetics, cryotherapy, sunscreens.

Campbell de Morgan spot (cherry angioma; haemangioma)

Clinical features Multiple, small bright red spots (Fig. 151), often familial, on trunk of middle-aged and elderly.

Treatment None; diathermy.

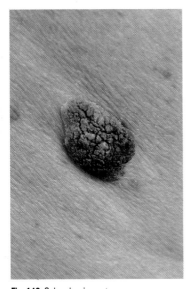

Fig. 148 Seborrhoeic wart.

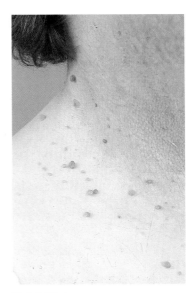

Fig. 149 Skin tags.

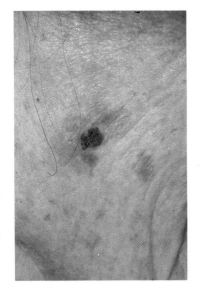

Fig. 150 Solar lentigo/seborrhoeic wart.

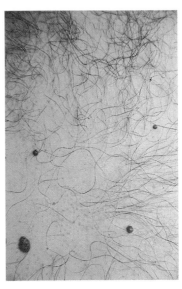

Fig. 151 Campbell de Morgan angiomas.

Solar keratosis (actinic keratosis)

Aetiology — Chronic exposure to UVL.

Clinical features — Commoner in the fair-skinned or expatriates, in middle to old age. It affects the backs of hands forehead, scalp, temples, nose, cheeks and ears, with rough, adherent crusts on an erythematous base (Fig. 152).

Treatment — Curettage and trichloracetic acid; cryotherapy; 5-fluorouracil cream for multiple lesions.

Bowen's disease

Aetiology — Previous exposure to UVL/or arsenic, pre-invasive intraepidermal carcinoma.

Clinical features — Appearing anywhere on the skin or mucosal surfaces as asymptomatic, erythematous, well-demarcated, scaly patches (Fig. 153). Ulceration suggests invasive growth.

Treatment — Surgical excision; cryotherapy; 5-fluorouracil.

Keratoacanthoma

Clinical features — Occurs in middle to old age, mainly on face or dorsum of hands. A flesh-coloured papule enlarges rapidly over 8–10 weeks with a central keratin-filled crater (Fig. 154). Spontaneous involution leaves depressed scar.

Treatment — Surgical excision.

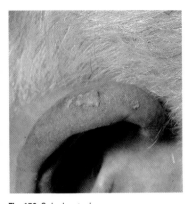

Fig. 152 Solar keratosis.

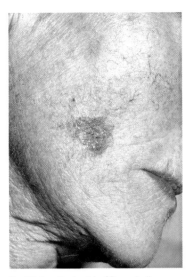

Fig. 153 Localized patch of Bowen's disease on the face.

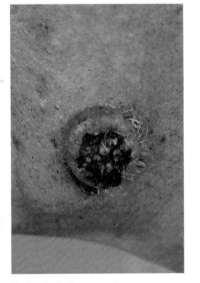

Fig. 154 Typical keratoacanthoma.

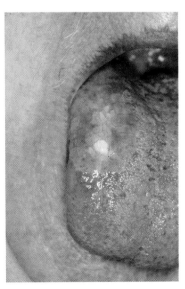

Fig. 155 Leukoplakia (carcinoma in situ). Well-demarcated white patches on tongue.

Basal cell carcinoma (BCC)

Aetiology Chronic cutaneous sun-damage or exposure to arsenicals or radiotherapy.

Clinical features Commonest cutaneous malignancy. It occurs in middle to old age, usually on the head and neck. The lesion classically begins as a raised, pearly or translucent papule with telangiectasia, central ulceration and a typical rolled edge (Fig. 156). It may be pigmented, multifocal or sclerotic/morphoeic (Fig. 158). Fibrosing or penetrating BCC may erode underlying tissues.

Treatment Surgical excision; radiotherapy; curettage and cautery. Superficial multi-focal BCCs are sometimes treated with aggressive cryotherapy.

Squamous cell carcinoma (SCC)

Aetiology Exposure to sunlight. Industrial carcinogens and longstanding ulcers also predispose.

Clinical features May develop 'de novo' or on previously sun-damaged skin or with a background of solar keratosis, Bowen's disease or leukoplakia. The lesions begin as nodules on a firm indurated base, ulcerating as they enlarge (Fig. 157), commonly on the backs of hands and face, especially the lower lip and ear. Metastases are uncommon in the sun-induced type, but more frequent in 'de novo' SCC or on a background of Bowen's disease or leukoplakia (Fig. 155, p. 102).

Treatment Surgical excision.

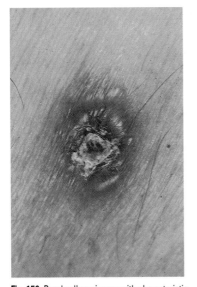

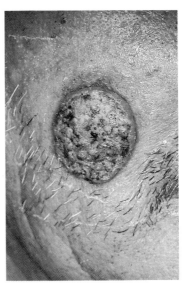

Fig. 156 Basal cell carcinoma with characteristic rolled, pearly edge.

Fig. 157 Squamous cell carcinoma of the face.

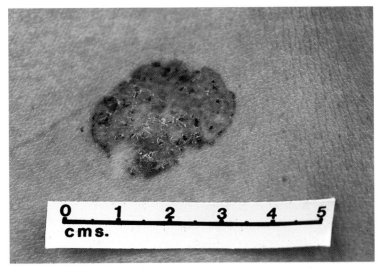

Fig. 158 Superficial multifocal pigmented BCC.

31 / **Melanoma**

Lentigo maligna

Aetiology   Intraepidermal, pre-invasive, malignant melanoma.

Clinical features   Appears in middle to old age as a flat brown stain with an irregular, well-demarcated edge, slowly enlarging with variable pigmentation. It most commonly affects the face. Nodular malignant melanoma may develop after many years (Fig. 159).

Treatment   Cryotherapy or superficial radiotherapy in the macular phase. Excision if small or nodular.

Malignant melanoma

Aetiology   Excessive exposure to sunlight.

Clinical features   Any 'new' mole or one which changes its character in adult life should be regarded as malignant melanoma until proved otherwise. Rapidly becoming one of the commonest form of cancer in those between the ages of 20–50 years. Prognosis deteriorates rapidly and early referral is obligatory. Superficial spreading melanoma starts as a slightly elevated irregular brown or black patch (Fig. 160). Nodule formation indicates a vertically invasive stage (Figs 161 & 162). *Nodular melanoma* has a worse prognosis. Melanoma under the nail may be mistaken for subungual haemorrhage.

Treatment   Early wide excision with block dissection of lymph nodes if involved.

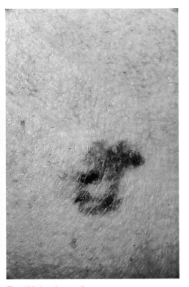

Fig. 159 Lentigo maligna.

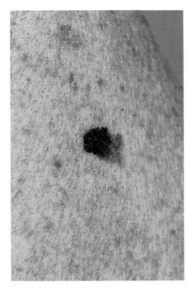

Fig. 160 Superficial spreading melanoma.

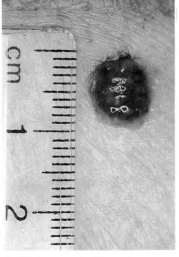

Fig. 161 Amelanotic (nodular) malignant melanoma.

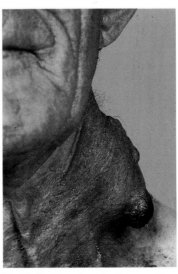

Fig. 162 Nodular malignant melanoma with lymphadenopathy.

32 / Contact dermatitis

Aetiology

Irritant contact dermatitis (ICD): may be *acute* (strong irritants) or *cumulative* (mild irritants e.g. detergents/solvents), with progression from *irritant reaction* (dryness/chapping) to dermatitis. Atopy is a predisposing factor.

Allergic CD (Figs 163–166): due to type IV (delayed) lymphocyte-mediated hypersensitivity. Common allergens include nickel, chromate, rubber chemicals, medicaments and cosmetics (preservatives/fragrance). Industrial allergens include epoxy, acrylate and phenol formaldehyde resins. Plant allergens include *Compositae, Primula obconica, Rhus* (poison oak/ivy) and various other woods and balsams.

Photo CD: may be allergic (e.g. musk ambrette), toxic (phytophotodermatitis) or simply light aggravated.

Clinical features

Hands and face, being in most contact with the environment, are the sites most commonly affected. The cause of the dermatitis may be obvious from the history, but patch testing is often necessary. Facial allergens may be volatile (airborne) or cosmetic. Medicament CD may be a complicating factor in stasis ulcers, chronic ear/eye disorders and in pruritus ani due to prolonged usage on damaged skin.

Treatment

Identify cause and advise on avoidance/protection. Soap substitute, e.g. aqueous cream, can be used to clean/wash; 'barrier' creams make hands easier to clean but afford no protection. Other treatments include: emollients, topical steroids in strengths appropriate to severity of eczema and, rarely, systemic steroids. Antihistamines can be used for symptomatic relief.

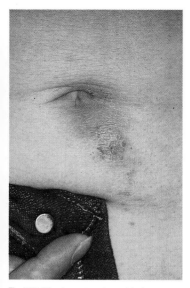

Fig. 163 Allergic contact dermatitis due to nickel jean stud.

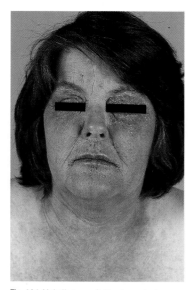

Fig. 164 Volatile type of allergic contact dermatitis due to phosphorous sesquisulphide in matches.

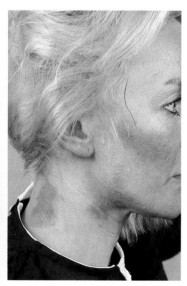

Fig. 165 Patchy erythema on neck due to nail varnish.

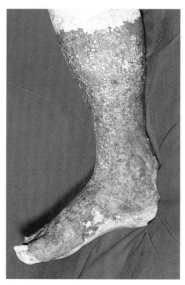

Fig. 166 Lower leg is an important site for medicament sensitivity.

33 / Hand eczema

Synonym	Hand dermatitis.
Aetiology	Constitutional or exogenous, frequently both, and impossible to differentiate on clinical appearances alone (Fig. 167). Atopics are more prone to irritant hand eczema.
Clinical features	***Constitutional patterns*** of hand eczema include: recurrent pompholyx; vesicular/hyperkeratotic hand eczema and hyperkeratotic hand eczema.

Exogenous patterns of hand eczema include:
1. Irritant patterns
   - 'Ring' eczema from wet work/detergents (Fig. 168).
   - 'Web' eczema/dorsum of hands from wet work.
   - 'Finger-tip' and 'palmar' patterns due to wet cloths, frictional factors, etc.
   - 'Patchy'/'discoid' patterns.
2. Allergic patterns
   - 'Non-specific'. Most cases, e.g. with perfumes, preservatives, etc., will be missed unless routine patch testing is performed.
   - 'Specific patterns', e.g. rubber glove dermatitis (Fig. 169), ring dermatitis and fingertip eczema.
   - Atopics may also develop type I *contact urticaria* or *protein contact dermatitis* from food handling and preparation.

Treatment   Identify the cause. Patch testing is helpful. Provide hand care advice, e.g. cotton-lined PVC gloves for wet work and frequent applications of emollients. Potent steroids with or without antibiotics can be used for for secondary infection. Atopics with a history of eczema should be given employment counselling.

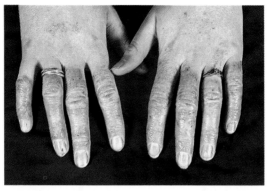

Fig. 167 Hand dermatitis: irritant and allergic factors frequently coexist.

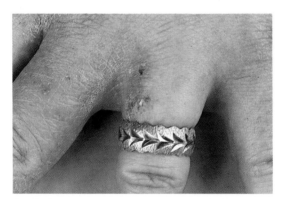

Fig. 168 'Ring' dermatitis—may be due to irritants, but occasionally associated with nickel allergy.

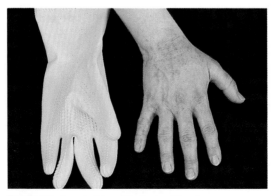

Fig. 169 Allergic contact dermatitis due to rubber gloves.

Pompholyx

Aetiology A common form of endogenous eczema. It may be a reaction to an active fungal infection of the feet. Ingested allergens (e.g. nickel in females) are sometimes implicated.

Clinical features A recurrent, intensely itchy, symmetrical eruption of the hands (and/or feet) with crops of clear vesicles on the sides of fingers and palms (Fig. 170). These may become confluent, producing large bullae. Secondary infection is common (Fig. 171). Skin subsequently becomes dry/fissured and desquamates.

Treatment
- Frequent potassium permanganate soaks initially.
- Potent topical steroids/antibacterial combinations.
- Antihistamines for symptomatic relief.
- Systemic steroids for severe attacks.
- Antibiotics if secondary infection.
- Treat athlete's foot if present.

Hyperkeratotic palmar eczema

Aetiology Uncommon constitutional eczema not related to atopy. Factors include friction and underlying hyperkeratotic or psoriasiform tendency.

Clinical features Usually affects middle-aged, with intensely itchy, hyperkeratotic patches of fissured eczema on palms. Rarely, there may be a few vesicles (Fig. 172).

Treatment Potent topical steroids, antipruritic antihistamines, soap substitutes/emollients, tar, avoidance of friction and superficial RXT.

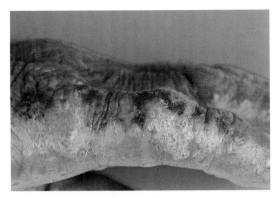

Fig. 170 Vesicular hand dermatitis (pompholyx).

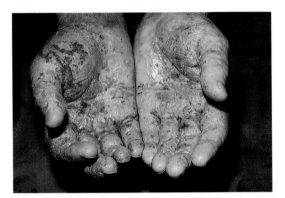

Fig. 171 Infected hand eczema.

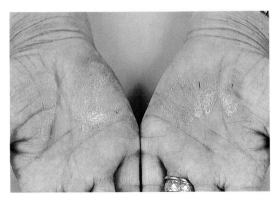

Fig. 172 Hyperkeratotic hand eczema.

Seborrhoeic eczema

Aetiology Unknown; not due to increased sebum production. Pityrosporum ovale/orbiculare infection may be important.

Clinical features **Infantile:** 'cradle cap' (p. 25); napkin (p. 17).
Adult: in young adults (usually men), it commonly involves scalp, ears, eyebrows, eyelids, nasolabial folds, central chest and pubic area. There are greasy scales on a background of erythema associated with generally greasy, easily irritated/intolerant skin (Figs 173 & 174). In the elderly, it is commonly intertriginous. Moist erythematous areas are often the sites of bacterial/candidal infection (Fig. 175).

Treatment Soap substitutes; weak topical steroids, steroid/antibiotic/antiseptic combinations; sulphur and salicylic acid cream, lithium succinate ointment, tar or imidazole shampoos, and steroid scalp applications.

Asteototic eczema

Aetiology Reduced lipids and water binding capacity of the stratum corneum leads to drying/cracking of the skin. The condition is aggravated by excess washing and low temperature/humidity. It is occasionally associated with malnutrition, general debility, diuretic therapy, myxoedema and renal failure.

Clinical features Common in old age; itchy, dry and scaly with reticulate cracks. It normally affects legs, but trunk and arms may be involved. Discoid eczema may coexist. Rarely, there may be an underlying malignancy.

Treatment Emollients, bath oils, fewer baths; weak topical steroids.

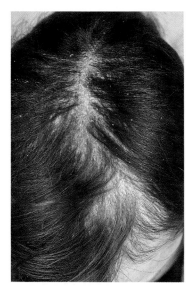

Fig. 173 Seborrhoeic dermatitis of scalp.

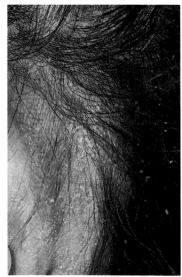

Fig. 174 Scalp margin and retro-auricular seborrhoeic dermatitis.

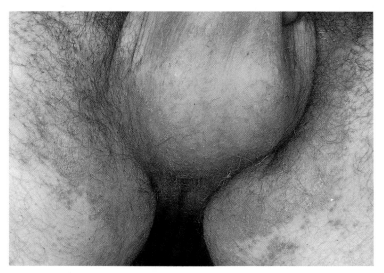

Fig. 175 Seborrhoeic dermatitis of the groin.

Discoid eczema

Synonym Nummular eczema.

Aetiology A constitutional pattern of eczema. The condition characteristically occurs in middle-aged men (executives), and stress, over-washing and low humidity, e.g. central heating, air-conditioning, car heaters, etc., may be important. Well-demarcated coin-shaped areas of eczema (Fig. 176), normally affect the extensor surfaces of limbs (Fig. 177), but with subsequent explosive spread to a more generalized pattern of eczema (Fig. 178). One or two solitary patches often pre-date the general eruption by some weeks or months. Pruritus may be intense. Lesions are often vesicular and exudative and may become secondarily infected. Discoid eczema may sometimes be associated with an 'extensor' pattern of atopic eczema and, rarely, with contact allergy, e.g. chromate.

Treatment Soap substitutes; a reduction in bathing; an increase in the humidity of surroundings. Treatments also include emollients, oral antihistamines, potent steroids or steroid/antibacterial combinations and antibiotics. Systemic steroids may sometimes be required, and tar may be of help in more chronic cases.

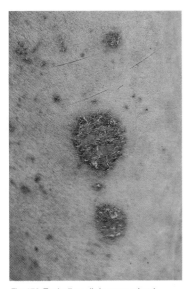

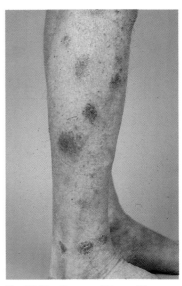

Fig. 176 Typically well-demarcated and exudative lesions of discoid eczema.

Fig. 177 Discoid eczema. This condition may sometimes be mistaken for a fungal infection.

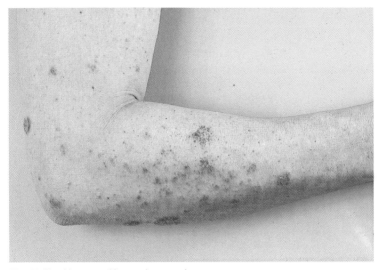

Fig. 178 Discoid eczema with secondary spread.

Stasis eczema and ulcers

Aetiology   Venous hypertension results from deep vein thrombosis or familial valvular incompetence, with incompetent, perforating veins leading to poor tissue perfusion/oxygenation and the development of stasis eczema and ulcers.

Clinical features   Usually seen in obese, middle aged women, with characteristic 'champagne bottle' leg. Skin changes usually start on the medial aspect of lower leg at site of perforating veins, as stasis pigmentation or liposclerosis. Oedema may become gross (elephantiasis nostras) (Fig. 179) or the leg may become progressively more fibrotic and sclerotic (Fig. 180) due to strangled microcirculation (atrophie blanche).

Complications   Ulceration can often follow minimal trauma with the 'atrophie blanche' type leg. Secondary infection is invariable, but normally only pathogenic bacteria (group A streptococci and *Staph. aureus*) require treatment. Streptococcal infection may cause cellulitis. Topical antibiotics frequently provoke allergic contact sensitization (Fig. 175, p. 114).

Treatment   Weight reduction; paste/compressive bandages; support stockings when ulcers are healed; rest with legs up. Oil helps scaly dry skin. Antiseptic solutions can be used to clean ulcers before applying simple dressings, e.g. paraffin gauze. Systemic antibiotics can be administered for secondary infection; moderate strength steroids for eczema. Surgery is required for varicosities/incompetent perforators.

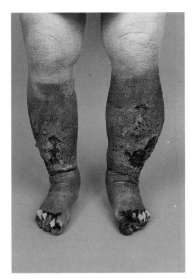

Fig. 179 Elephantiasis nostras.

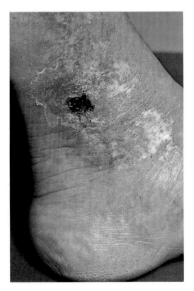

Fig. 180 'Atrophie blanche'.

35 / **Localized patterns of itch**

Lichen simplex (neurodermatitis)

Aetiology

A localized, sometimes eczematous response to constant rubbing; often partly habit and frequently triggered by stress.

Clinical features

Several characteristic patterns:
- women—the nape of neck, side of neck and vulva
- men—the ankle/shin (Fig. 181), scrotum and perianal area (Fig. 182).
- both sexes—the elbow and central palms.

The lichenified lesions are usually solitary and well-demarcated, more diffuse on the scrotum and the perianal area, due to repeated scratching and rubbing (Fig. 183).

Treatment

Potent topical steroids, tar or tar paste bandages, sedative antihistamines, occasionally intralesional steroids.

Pruritus ani

Aetiology

Predisposing factors include haemorrhoids, fissures, irritation from mucous or faecal leak, sweat/maceration, contact dermatitis, threadworm infection (in children).

Clinical features

Lichen simplex, maceration, fissuring or bacterial/candidal intertrigo (Fig. 184).

Treatment

Treat underlying or complicating factors. Soap substitutes, mild/moderate corticosteroid/antiseptic preparations; sedative antihistamines.

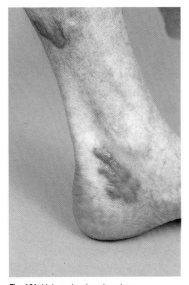

Fig. 181 Lichen simplex chronicus.

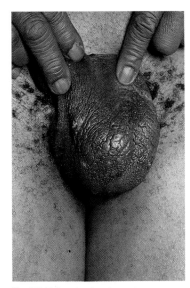

Fig. 182 Lichen simplex of scrotum.

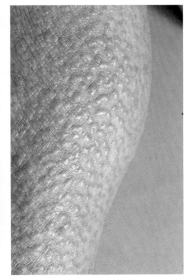

Fig. 183 Pebbly lichenification from constant rubbing.

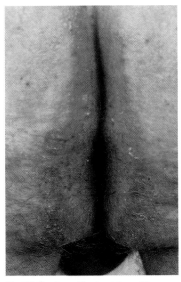

Fig. 184 Pruritus ani/perianal dermatitis.

Prurigo

Clinical features 'Prurigo' is a term used to describe any localized skin abnormality where the principal symptom is itch. Lesions include excoriations, prurigo nodules and localized areas of lichen simplex.

'Cape prurigo': a common pattern in the elderly (Fig. 185). Dry skin and low serum iron are important factors.

'Tycoon scalp': a characteristic pattern of excoriation of the scalp, mainly affecting businessmen and frequently associated with stress. Folliculitis and seborrhoeic dermatitis may be initiating factors (Fig. 186).

Subacute prurigo: mainly affects the extensor aspects of limbs in women but more diffuse patterns also occur.

Nodular prurigo: an intransigent pattern of prurigo with intensely pruriginous nodules separated by areas of normal skin. It mainly affects the extensor aspects of limbs (Fig. 187).

Treatment 'Cape' prurigo often responds to simple emollients, iron replacement therapy and sedative antihistamines. Crotamiton/hydrocortisone cream is also helpful. Other patterns of prurigo are very intransigent and respond poorly to treatment. The itch/scratch/itch habit is difficult to break. Potent steroids, occlusive tar paste bandages, sedative antihistamines and, occasionally, intralesional steroids are required.

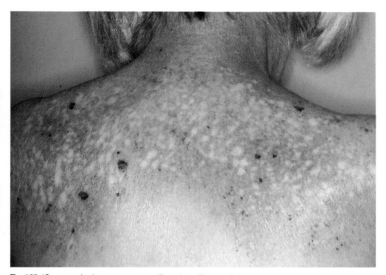

Fig. 185 'Cape prurigo': a common manifestation of iron deficiency in the elderly.

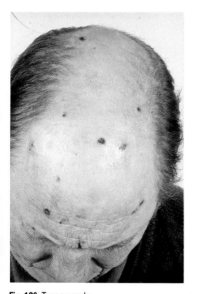

Fig. 186 Tycoon scalp.

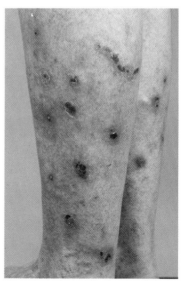

Fig. 187 Nodular prurigo.

36 / **Leg ulcers**

Aetiology
- Secondary to venous hypertension (p. 117).
- Secondary to arterial disease. Ulceration may follow arterial thrombosis, atherosclerosis, vasculitis or small vessel disease such as that associated with rheumatoid arthritis and diabetes. Hypertension is an important complicating factor.
- Neuropathic ulcers occur in diabetes (Fig. 188), alcoholics and in leprosy. They particularly involve the foot/lower leg. Secondary infection also often plays a part.
- Malignancy—a progressive, non-healing or 'atypical' leg ulcer should raise the question of a basal cell or squamous cell carcinoma.
- Other rare causes include sickle cell disease, spherocytosis, cryoglobulinaemia and tertiary syphilis (Fig. 189).

Clinical features

Venous ulcers: often large and messy, and usually associated with other signs of venous hypertension (p. 117).

Arterial ulcers: more often affect the foot and lateral aspects of the legs. Peripheral pulses may be diminished or absent and pain is a constant feature, especially at night or when dressings are too tight. The ulcers have a characteristic 'punched out' appearance (Fig. 190) with a well-defined regular edge.

Treatment

Treatment of venous ulcers is discussed on p. 117. In arterial disease, treatment is generally unsatisfactory since the underlying cause of the ischaemia is rarely reversible. Hypertension should be controlled, but N.B. betablockers reduce tissue perfusion. Appropriate antibiotics should be used for secondary infection; intravascular abnormalities should be corrected where possible. Adequate analgesia is important, and dressings should be simple and non-constricting.

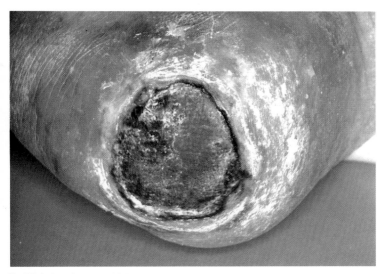

Fig. 188 Ischaemic neuropathic/pressure ulcer on heel of diabetic.

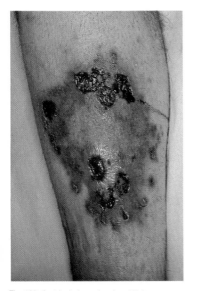

Fig. 189 Atypical ulceration (syphilis).

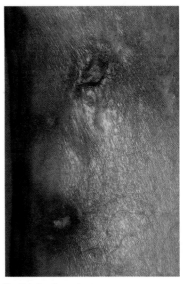

Fig. 190 Small punched out arterial ulcers.

37 / Skin manifestations of internal malignancy

Acanthosis nigricans

Aetiology   Normally underlying adenocarcinoma of stomach, breast or lung, but benign and genetic forms also exist.

Clinical features   Thick, ridged, warty plaques give a velvety appearance in the axillae (Fig. 191) and groin. Heavily pigmented skin is seen (may antedate the clinical appearance of carcinoma by 3 or 4 years). Benign forms occasionally occur both as genetic disease and as a complication of endocrine disease and obesity (Fig. 192).

Treatment   Treatment of the underlying condition may lead to resolution of the skin changes, but these may recur if the carcinoma spreads or undergoes metastasis.

Acquired ichthyosis

Aetiology   Normally associated with underlying reticuloses, e.g. Hodgkin's disease or mycosis fungoides. Occasionally drugs, malabsorption and malnutrition are involved.

Clinical features   Itchy, dry and scaly skin (Fig. 193). There may be hyperkeratosis of the palms and soles.

Treatment   Treat the underlying disorder. Emollients, antipruritics and antihistamines

Other skin manifestations of internal malignancy

Erythema gyratum repens, migratory thrombophlebitis (Fig. 194), and generalized pruritus are also in this category of disorder. Other recorded associations are less reliably attributed to underlying malignant disease.

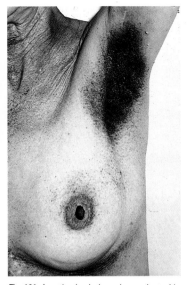

Fig. 191 Acanthosis nigricans in a patient with underlying malignancy.

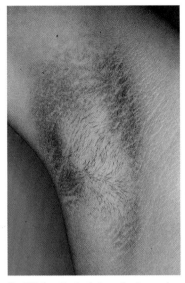

Fig. 192 Acanthosis nigricans (benign type).

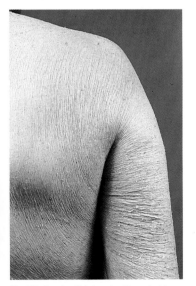

Fig. 193 Acquired ichthyosis with underlying lymphoma.

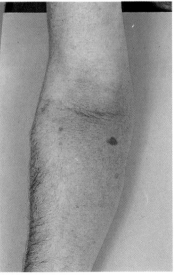

Fig. 194 Migratory thrombophlebitis.

Dermatomyositis

Aetiology An autoimmune disease. In those over 40, approximately half the cases will have an underlying carcinoma of lung, ovary, breast, uterus or stomach, but there is no such association in childhood.

Clinical features A characteristic violaceous rash associated with myositis. There is also often a myopathy, and if this involves the respiratory muscles, the disease can be life-threatening. Other associations include arthralgia, Raynaud's phenomenon, fever and prostration. Calcinosis cutis is common in the childhood form. Erythema, fine scaling and telangiectasia affect the face with heliotrope discolouration of the upper eyelids (Fig. 195). Violaceous plaques occur over the knuckles, and cuticles become thick and ragged with prominent nail-fold telangiectasia (Fig. 196). Oedema of the hands and face is common. The rash may generalize.

Treatment High-dose steroids are required. Bed-rest, splints and support for involved muscles and joints, and general supportive treatment are important. Seek and treat underlying carcinoma.

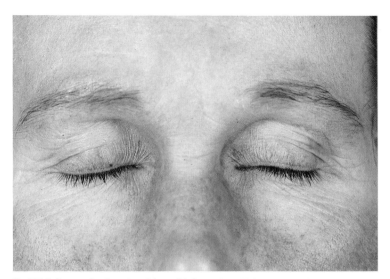

Fig. 195 Heliotrope discolouration of the eyelids in a patient with immune type dermatomyositis.

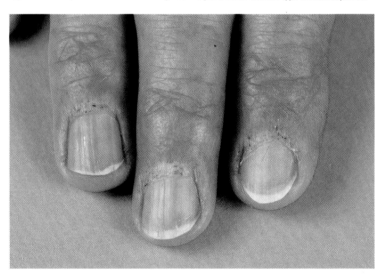

Fig. 196 Nail fold thromboses in a patient with dermatomyositis.

38 / Autoimmune diseases

Vitiligo

Aetiology One of a group of organ-specific autoimmune diseases with antimelanocyte antibodies.

Clinical features Well-defined oval or irregular depigmented areas (symmetrical and a few mm to several cm in size) affecting axillae, groins, genitalia, dorsum of hands and face (Figs 197 & 198). Hair in the affected areas may also become white. The involved skin tends to burn on sun exposure but is otherwise asymptomatic. Other organ-specific autoimmune diseases may coexist, e.g. thyroid disease, pernicious anaemia, diabetes mellitus and alopecia areata in both patients and their families (Fig. 199).

Treatment Not universally successful. Repigmentation may sometimes be induced with intermittent potent, topical steroids or PUVA. Cosmetic camouflage and sunscreens can be helpful.

Halo naevus

Aetiology Localized form of vitiligo

Clinical features An area of depigmentation surrounding a small pigmented cellular naevus (Fig. 200). The central naevus usually disappears over several weeks and repigmentation may then occur, or a leukodermic area persist. Some patients develop vitiligo.

Treatment Sunscreens to protect vitiliginous area.

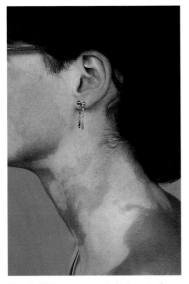

Fig. 197 Vitiligo contrasted with islands of normally pigmented skin.

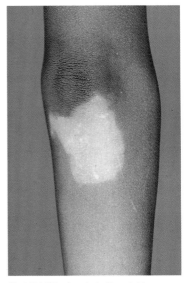

Fig. 198 Vitiligo in a dark skinned girl.

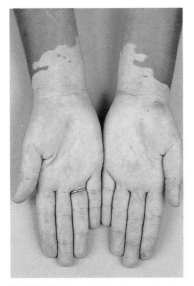

Fig. 199 Vitiligo in a patient with co-existent Addison's disease.

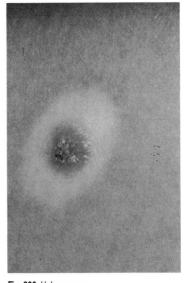

Fig. 200 Halo naevus.

Scleroderma

Synonyms Systemic sclerosis; acrosclerosis; morphoea.

Aetiology Unknown but thought to be autoimmune.

Clinical features There are three principal types of scleroderma.
- A *multisystem* disease (*acrosclerosis*) commonly affects women. Raynaud's phenomenon is a frequent presenting symptom. The skin of the hands and face is hard and tightly bound down. The fingers become tapered, flexed and shiny with loss of finger pulps (sclerodactyly) (Fig. 201). There may be nail-fold thromboses and fingertip ulceration. The face becomes mask-like with pinching of the nose and mouth. Telangiectasia and calcium deposits in the fingers are common. The gastrointestinal tract, liver, kidneys, joints and lungs may also be involved.
- A more *progressive* form (*progressive systemic sclerosis*) affects both sexes equally. Morbidity and mortality are significant.
- *Localized cutaneous scleroderma* (*morphoea*) normally affects young adults, and women more than men. Ill-defined purplish, sclerotic plaques develop insidiously on the trunk and elsewhere, often symmetrically and progressing slowly over a matter of months/years (Fig. 202). Special variants include 'coup de sabre' (parietofrontal), linear (Fig. 203) and generalized forms.

Treatment Always very disappointing. Steroids, penicillamine, vitamin E and immunosuppressants have been tried.

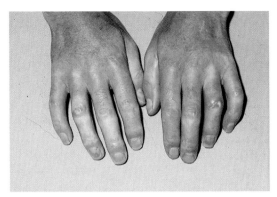

Fig. 201 Acrosclerosis.

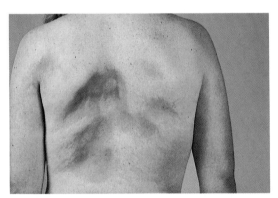

Fig. 202 Localized morphoea.

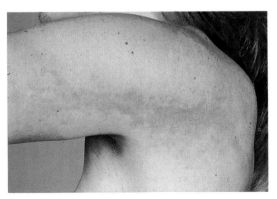

Fig. 203 Linear morphoea.

39 / Systemic lupus erythematosus (SLE)

Aetiology Genetic predisposition to this and other autoimmune diseases. Virus infections and pregnancy may act as triggers. Drugs, e.g. hydrallazine and procainamide, can sometimes provoke an SLE-like syndrome.

Clinical features A multisystem disease affecting women more than men. The skin, joints, kidneys, lungs, CNS and other organs may all be involved. Lymphopenia and thrombocytopenia are both common. There is often an element of photosensitivity or an eruption confined to light-exposed areas. This may be 'discoid-LE-like' (p. 75) or quite non-specific consisting simply of erythema or a discrete maculopapular eruption (Fig. 204). The classical pattern consists of a symmetrical patchy erythema, sometimes with scaling, telangiectasia and induration, occurring on the cheeks and bridge of the nose producing a typical 'butterfly' rash. The hands are also often affected and there may be vasculitis (p. 65), persistent non-itchy weals, livedo (Fig. 205) and chilblain-like lesions during the winter. Nail-fold infarcts and splinter haemorrhages occur in association with Raynaud's phenomenon (p. 131). There may be general symptoms including arthralgia, malaise and fever. Alopecia (Fig. 206) occurs in up to 50% of patients.

Treatment Avoidance of exacerbating factors, e.g. cold and sunshine, and symptomatic treatment may be sufficient. Systemic steroids and immunosuppressants are usually required for more severe disease.

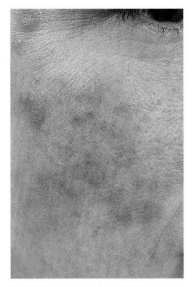

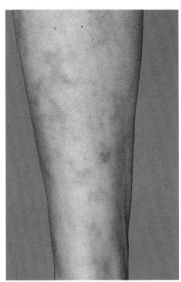

Fig. 204 Maculopapular-type LE of face.

Fig. 205 Livedo reticularis (SLE).

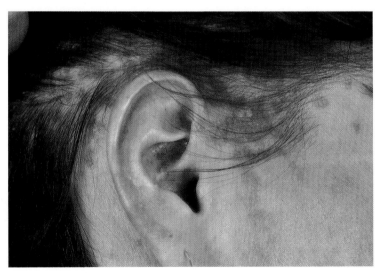

Fig. 206 Discoid LE-like lesions and scarring alopecia in a patient with SLE.

40 / Side-effects of topical steroids

Adverse effects of topical steroids depend on:
- potency of preparation
- length of use
- site of use.

Aetiology Steroids inhibit dermal collagen synthesis.

Clinical features **Atrophy:** thinning of skin occurs with long-term use of potent topical steroids. Affected areas are erythematous and fragile with telangiectasia (Fig. 207).

Striae: commonly seen in axillae and groins; initial 'stretch marks' are purple and later become white (Fig. 208).

Purpura or bruising: may arise following minimal trauma.

Tinea or impetigo incognita: topical steroids may mask the characteristic appearance of fungal or bacterial infections (p. 97)

Perioral dermatitis. (p. 67)

Adrenal suppression: Application of potent topical steroids in large quantities (50–100 g/week) or under occlusion may lead to temporary suppression of pituitary-adrenal function. This is particularly important in young children.

Granuloma gluteale infantum: occurs in infants a few months old who have received topical steroid applications for napkin rash. Small, often multiple, red-brown nodules develop anywhere within the napkin area. Nodules resolve slowly once the application of topical steroids is stopped (p. 16).

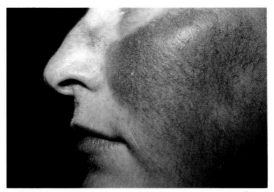

Fig. 207 Steroid-induced telangiectasia.

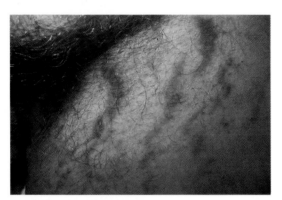

Fig. 208 Striae from topical steroids.

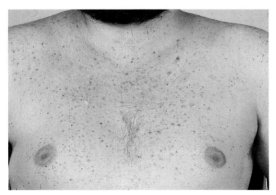

Fig. 209 Steroid acne folliculitis—a consequence of high dose systemic steroid therapy.

41 / **Dermal reactions**

Sarcoidosis

Aetiology Unknown. A multisystem, granulomatous disease.

Clinical features **Erythema nodosum** (p. 63).
Lupus pernio (Fig. 210): indurated, soft, blue-red plaques affect nose, ears, fingers, cheeks.
Papulonodular: firm, blue-red papules, nodules or plaques affect the face, trunk and extensor surfaces of limbs. Annular lesions also occur.
Scar sarcoid: existing scars may become infiltrated.

Treatment Oral steroids if systemic symptoms warrant.

Annular erythema

Aetiology Often idiopathic. Drugs, infections and carcinoma have been implicated. Variants include erythema chronicum migrans (tick bite), erythema gyratum repens (underlying carcinoma) and erythema marginatum (active rheumatic fever).

Clinical features Small, pink papules enlarge slowly to form ring or polycyclic patterns with central clearing (Fig. 211). They may be solitary or multiple, lasting weeks/months.

Treatment Symptomatic.

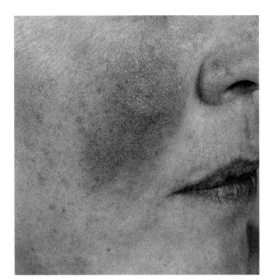

Fig. 210 Lupus pernio.

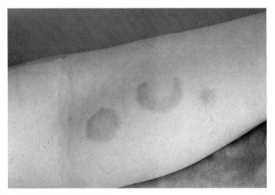

Fig. 211 Annular erythema.

Granuloma annulare

Aetiology   Unknown. It may be associated with diabetes mellitus.

Clinical features   Commonly affects adolescents. Solitary or multiple firm, smooth, skin-coloured or violaceous papules appear on the dorsum of hands/feet (Fig. 212), fingers, ankles, elbows and elsewhere. Typically they progress into annular lesions. Most resolve spontaneously within 1–2 yr.

Treatment   None. Potent steroids with occlusion; intralesional corticosteroids rarely.

Necrobiosis lipoidica

Aetiology   Unknown. Some cases are associated with diabetes.

Clinical features   A reddish-brown, slowly enlarging plaque with shiny, yellow, atrophic centre (Fig. 213) classically involving the front of the shins. Lesions show telangiectasia and some eventually ulcerate. Differential diagnosis: granuloma annulare, basal cell carcinoma.

Treatment   Test for diabetes. Potent topical steroids (with occlusion) are of some value.

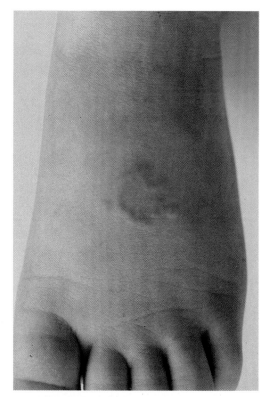

Fig. 212 Granuloma annulare.

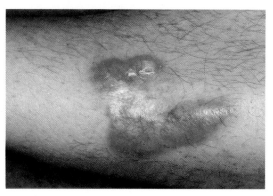

Fig. 213 Necrobiosis lipoidica.

Keloids/hypertrophic scars

Aetiology Excess proliferation of dermal collagen. Risk is increased with tension, infection or foreign material. There is occasionally a family history. Hypertrophic scars commoner in Negroes.

Clinical features Firm, raised, smooth, pink (or in Negroes brown) plaques or nodules develop 4–6 weeks after skin trauma, particularly on the ear lobe (after ear-piercing; Fig. 214), and on the upper back, shoulders, neck and presternal areas. Keloids tend to be irregular and to spread beyond the original injury.

Treatment Intralesional steroids or potent topical steroids under occlusion may help.

Xanthomatosis (hyperlipidaemias)

Aetiology Localized cutaneous deposits of lipid. The condition may be primary or secondary to diabetes, myxoedema, pancreatitis and nephrotic syndrome.

Xanthelasma: symmetrical, firm, flat, yellow plaques affecting the upper and lower eyelids (Fig. 216). There is usually no lipid abnormality; some have type II hyperlipidaemia with raised cholesterol levels and a positive family history.

Xanthomata: firm, yellowish nodules over the knees, elbows (Fig. 217), heels and buttocks. Tendon xanthomas occur in types II and III hyperlipidaemia.

Eruptive xanthomata: small, yellow or red-brown papules occurring on the buttocks and extensor surfaces of the limbs; characteristic in type I and V lipidaemias but also common in type IV hyperlipidaemia.

Treatment Treat underlying hyperlipidaemia.

Dermatofibroma

A localized fibrotic tissue response to insect bites or other trauma (Fig. 215).

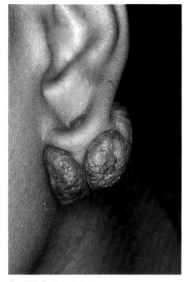

Fig. 214 Ear lobe keloid.

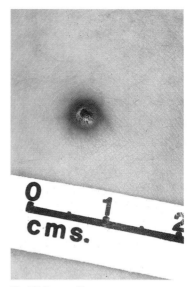

Fig. 215 Dermatofibroma.

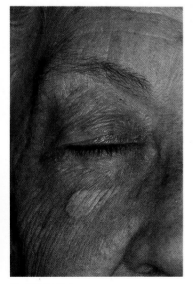

Fig. 216 Xanthelasma.

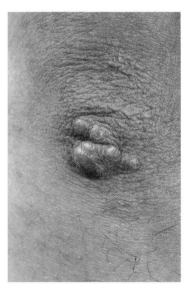

Fig. 217 Tuberous xanthoma.

Lichen planus

Clinical features   Mucous membrane lesions (Fig. 218) occur in 50% of cases but may occur in isolation. Candidiasis, secondary syphilis, leukoplakia must be differentiated.

Treatment   Symptomatic.

Geographic tongue

Clinical features   Benign, inflammatory disorder of unknown aetiology, usually asymptomatic. Multiple smooth, erythematous patches migrate in a map-like pattern on the dorsum of the tongue.

Treatment   None.

Recurrent aphthae

Clinical features   Common disorder of buccal mucosae, tongue, and gingival folds. Small, erythematous pustules rapidly break down to form painful shallow ulcers (Fig. 219) which heal in 7–10 days.

Treatment   Symptomatic; tetracycline mouthwash.

Black hairy tongue

Clinical features   May follow antibiotics and cytotoxics. The elongated papillae ('hair') may be yellow-brown or black.

Treatment   None.

Leukoplakia

Clinical features   Small, discrete, white patches or more extensive, leathery plaques on an atrophic erythematous base (Fig. 155, p. 102). Tobacco smoking and recurrent trauma predispose. Risk of malignant change (p. 103).

Treatment   Excision or cryotherapy.

Pemphigus

See page 81 (Fig. 220).

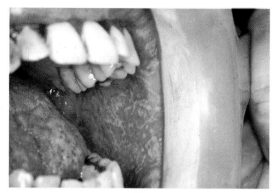

Fig. 218 Bluish-white lace-like striae of oral lichen planus.

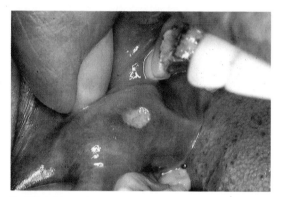

Fig. 219 Aphthous ulcer.

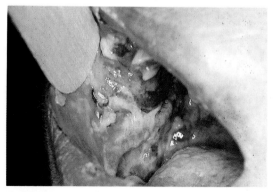

Fig. 220 Mucosal pemphigus.

43 / **Nails**

Onychogryphosis

Aetiology Age, trauma and ill-fitting shoes predispose.

Clinical features Usually affects the great toenails. Hypertrophy progresses to typical 'ram's horn' (Fig. 221).

Treatment Regular chiropody.

Onycholysis

Aetiology Causes include trauma (both physical and chemical), infection, psoriasis, eczema, poor circulation, photosensitivity to certain drugs, e.g. tetracyclines, and thyroid disease (Fig. 222).

Clinical features Lifting of the nail plate distally. A secondary pseudomonas infection may develop.

Treatment Reduce trauma. Keep nails short and dry.

Onychomycosis

Aetiology Usually *Trichophyton rubrum/T. mentagraphytes*.

Clinical features White or yellowish discolouration. The nail becomes thickened with subungual hyperkeratosis, splinter haemorrhages and onycholysis (Fig. 223).

Treatment Griseofulvin: 6 months for fingernails, 12–18 months for toenails. Terbinafine: 3 months for nails.

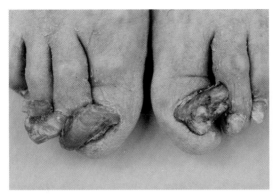

Fig. 221 Onychogryphosis.

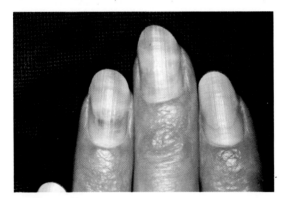

Fig. 222 Onycholysis.

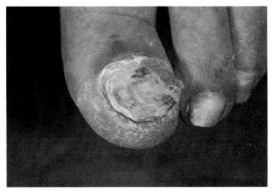

Fig. 223 Onychomycosis.

44 / **Nails in dermatological conditions**

Psoriasis

Clinical features The nails may be involved in the absence of psoriasis elsewhere with pitting, onycholysis (Fig. 224), subungual hyperkeratosis, yellowing/thickening and splinter haemorrhages.

Treatment Generally unrewarding.

Lichen planus

Clinical features Nail changes can occur in the absence of lesions elsewhere. It presents with increased longitudinal striations of nail plate, producing ridging and splitting. The nail plate becomes thinned and may progress to atrophy with scarring (Fig. 225) or even permanent destruction. The cuticle may grow over the base of the nail and attach to the nail plate.

Treatment Rarely, intralesional or systemic steroids.

Alopecia areata

Clinical features The nail plate becomes dull and roughened, with small, fine, regular pitting.

Treatment No specific treatment.

Eczema

Clinical features Nail changes can occur in any type of eczema, but are more often seen in atopic eczema. Several changes occur including: coarse pitting, transverse irregular ridging (Fig. 226), and shedding.

Treatment Treatment of the underlying eczema.

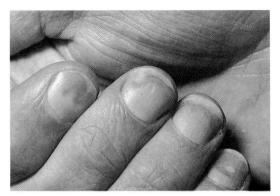

Fig. 224 Onycholysis and wax spots (psoriasis).

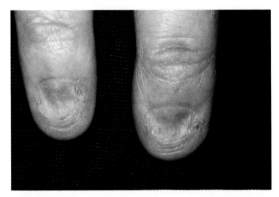

Fig. 225 Atrophy and scarring of the nail plate (lichen planus).

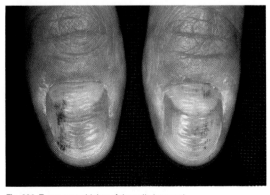

Fig. 226 Transverse ridging of the nails (eczema).

Lichen planus

Clinical features Characteristic mauve papules with fine lacework of white striae occur on the penile shaft, glans, and prepuce in men (Fig. 227), and in women, on the inner surface of the labia. Annular forms may also occur. Affected areas are frequently pruritic. Symptoms may occur with no evidence of lichen planus elsewhere. Treatment is symptomatic. (See also p. 51.)

Lichen sclerosus et atrophicus

Clinical features Uncommon (? autoimmune) disease mainly affecting women. Ivory-white or violaceous areas occur on the perianal and vulval regions with 'cigarette paper' atrophy. There may be follicular plugging, erosions and fissuring. In males, the glans penis and foreskin may be involved, leading to phimosis or meatal stricture (Fig. 228). Dyspareunia, soreness and pruritus often cause distress. The condition is potentially premalignant (in women).

Treatment No specific therapy known. Hydrocortisone/antiseptic creams for symptomatic relief; potent topical steroids initially and for phimosis or meatal strictures; 2% testosterone proprionate is also said to help. Surgery may be necessary.

Psoriasis

Clinical features Well-defined smooth, erythematous plaques on genitalia (Fig. 229). Important to differentiate from erythroplasia of Queyrak (Bowen's disease). (See also p. 45.)

Treatment Mild—moderate steroid/antibacterial creams.

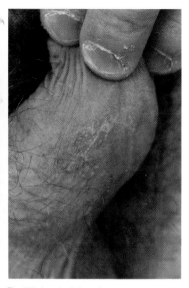

Fig. 227 Annular lichen planus.

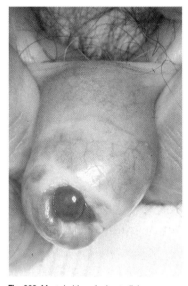

Fig. 228 Meatal phimosis due to lichen sclerosis et atrophicus.

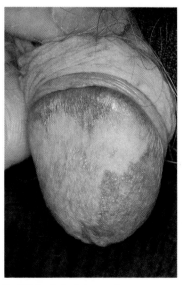

Fig. 229 Psoriasis of glans penis.

Alopecia areata

Aetiology   An organ-specific autoimmune disease.

Clinical features   Characterized by sudden hair loss in discrete, discoid patches (Fig. 230). Spontaneous regrowth often occurs in those with limited disease, although the new hair may initially be white. The condition occasionally progresses to involve the whole scalp (Fig. 231) or body. At the periphery of patches, diagnostic exclamation mark hairs are seen (Fig. 232). There may be associated fine pitting of the nails.

Treatment   Reassurance and wait for spontaneous regrowth. Topical or intralesional steroids, topical irritants (e.g. Dithranol), ultraviolet light/PUVA and contact sensitization may help. Topical 2% minoxidil solution may help those with localized patches. Wigs are an option.

Scarring alopecia

Aetiology   A result of destruction of hair follicles in, e.g. discoid lupus erythematosus, lichen planus, scleroderma, burns, infections and radiodermatitis.

Clinical features   Atrophic scalp with absent hair follicles. Once hair is lost regrowth never occurs. (See pp. 76 & 134.)

Management   Treatment of the underlying condition; wigs.

Male pattern baldness (androgenetic alopecia)

Aetiology   Genetically determined, androgen-sensitive pattern of hair loss.

Clinical features   Mainly affects men with early bi-temporal recession (Fig. 233) and loss of hair from vertex, progressing to more extensive patterns of baldness.

Treatment   None. Topical 2% minoxidil may reduce the loss and/or stimulate some short-term hair gain.

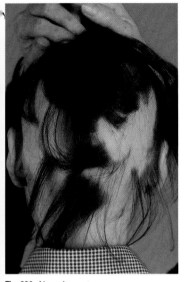

Fig. 230 Alopecia areata.

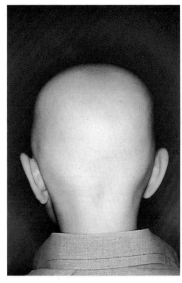

Fig. 231 Alopecia totalis.

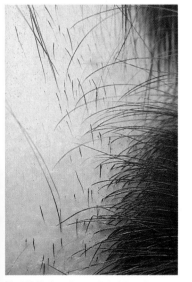

Fig. 232 Exclamation marks hair in active alopecia areata.

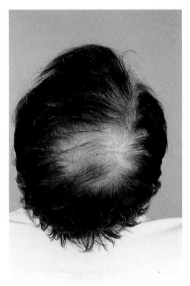

Fig. 233 Bi-temporal recession and early androgenic pattern hair loss.

47 / Human immunodeficiency virus (HIV) syndrome

Synonym	The acquired immunodeficiency syndrome (AIDS).
Aetiology	The results of infection with a human T-cell lymphotopic virus (HTLV III). AIDS is defined as a major disease indicative of defect in cell-mediated immunity for which no other cause other than HIV infection can be found.

Clinical features   HIV infection has four stages:

1. Acute infections—often asymptomatic or 'glandular fever-like' illness.
2. Prolonged asymptomatic/latent period of months to years.
3. Persistent generalized lymphadenopathy.
4. Symptomatic disease with progressive impairment of immune function:
   - constitutional disease, e.g. AIDS related complex (ARC).
   - neurological disease especially HIV *encephalopathy*.
   - secondary infections especially protozoal, viral, mycobacterial, fungal, etc.
   - *malignancies* e.g. Kaposi's sarcoma, non-Hodgkins lymphoma.
   - other conditions.

Cutaneous manifestations

Transient maculopapular or urticarial rash: may occur during acute HIV infection.

Seborrhoeic dermatitis (Fig. 234) and a papulopruritic eruption (itchy folliculitis) are common.

Kaposi's sarcoma: a multifocal endothelial cell neoplasm seen in a substantial minority of (especially homosexual) patients with AIDS. Reddish-brown or purple macules, nodules or plaques develop, often in skin creases or on nose or hard palate (Fig. 235).

Infections such as herpes zoster, herpes simplex, candidiasis, viral warts, molluscum contagiosum, fungal diseases and infections with exotic organisms such as cryptococcus, histoplasma, etc., occur secondary to immune dysfunction and may be both atypical and severe.

(*cont. on p. 155*)

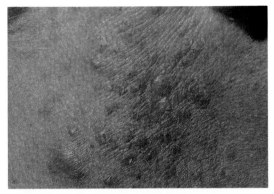

Fig. 234 Exacerbation of seborrhoeic dermatitis/psoriasis in a patient with AIDS.

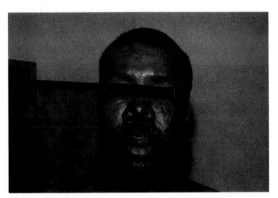

Fig. 235 Facial Kaposi's sarcoma.

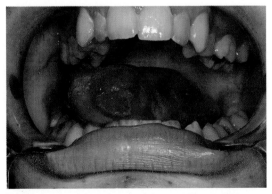

Fig. 236 Severe aphthous ulceration in haemophiliac with AIDS.

Oral hairy leukoplakia (associated with Epstein-Barr virus): presents as asymptomatic, vertically-ribbed keratinized plaques on the lateral borders of the tongue.

Bacterial angiomatosis

Drug eruption: common in patients with AIDS. ***Other associations*** include xeroderma, eosinophilic folliculitis, thrombocytopenic purpura, worsening of psoriasis, widespread granuloma annulare, demodicosis, prurigo, gingivitis, angular stomatitis, extensive pityriasis versicolor, severe aphthosis (Fig. 236, p. 154), worsening of eczema, vasculitis, norwegian scabies and the development of long eyelashes.

Treatment   Refer to specialist centres.

Index

Index